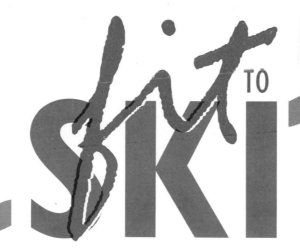

fit to SKI

• TONY WILSON •

Photographs by Roddy Paine

Cartoons by Stephen Ward

British Library Cataloguing in Publication Data
Fit to Ski
   1. Skiers. Physical fitness. Exercise
   I. Wilson, Tony
   613.711

   ISBN 0–340–52961–X

First published 1990

Typeset by Gecko Ltd, Bicester Oxon.
Printed in Great Britain for Hodder and Stoughton Educational, a
division of Hodder and Stoughton Ltd, by Martins of Berwick.

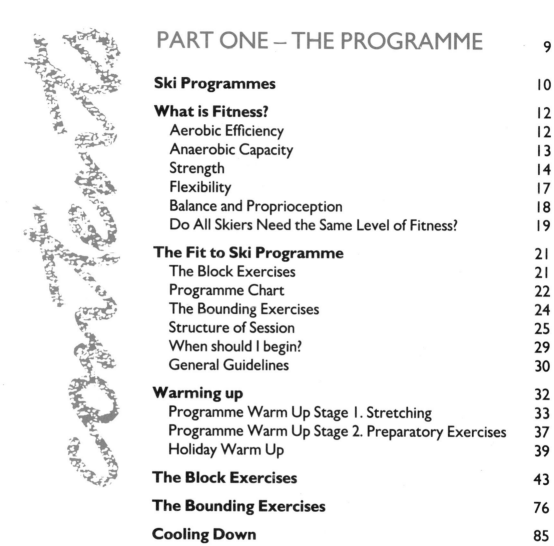

PART ONE – THE PROGRAMME 9

PART TWO: SKIING INJURIES – MANAGEMENT AND PREVENTION 87

Skiing has undergone an unprecedented rise in popularity in this country over the past decade. Increasingly people are taking more than one holiday each year and an extravagance once limited to all but the rich few now attracts more than 700,000 British skiers per season.

But it has grown into more than just a sport. It has developed around it an entire subculture with its own fashions and hype, its own stars and hangers-on, even its own language; so much so that in many ways it is now as much a part of the social calendar as it is a physical activity. A more dramatic change from the peasant strapping a rough-hewn plank of wood on both feet to ski down to the next village cannot be imagined. But there is a reason for this. Skiing is addictive. It is an expensive, frustrating, hazardous and at times maddening pastime, but once you have experienced the exhilaration of coasting down a pure white slope, the clear chill of the mountain air rushing past your cheeks and the unthinkably bright sun scorching down on you from a cold blue sky, once you have experienced the silence, then you are either unimpressed or hooked forever.

The choice of such a splendid holiday would tend to presume an effort on the part of the skier to enjoy it to the full. Sadly, however, in the majority of cases this effort does not appear to have been made. And yet behind the expensive multicoloured suits and shiny boots which only see daylight one or two weeks each year there lies a rigorous and exceptionally demanding physical activity. A skier's ability to cope with this, to enjoy skiing, develop exciting new skills, remain safe *and* look good on the slopes is directly related to his or her level of fitness.

Being fit enables you to perform more readily the complex series of skills that are demanded in skiing, it allows you to ski longer, to offset fatigue and so decrease the chance of injury, and it makes it possible for you to progress on to the more complicated manoeuvres and slopes more quickly. Quite simply, the fitter you are, the more you will enjoy it. Obviously, fitness is not the be all and end all of skiing; expert tuition, good equipment, a natural affinity for the sport are all useful to you, but fitness is the cornerstone around which they are built, the essential prerequisite without which the benefits of all other factors would be wasted. Believe me, with the best tuition, equipment and natural talent in the world, it is hard to marvel at the majesty of the mountains when your legs are aching and your heart and lungs are screaming with exhaustion. After all, to attempt to run the marathon without any prior training would generally evoke an incredulous response, yet people seem to think little of doing no preparation for skiing whatsoever and then launching themselves off the steepest slopes in the cosy belief that the skills and stamina which they achieved a year ago will be present to the same comforting degree this time. At best, this type of foolhardiness results in the gnawing ache of exhaustion, at worst appalling injury.

Even those who are far-sighted enough to do some preparation, all too often spend their time performing a vague mish-mash of exercises; going for the occasional run, doing a press-up or two and wasting endless hours sitting propped against the wall achieving little but sore legs and the distinct possibility of physical damage.

It is interesting to note that while companies pour massive amounts of funds into the research and development of new equipment, succeeding, as they have, in a quite startling decrease in the rate of casualties in skiing, one of the most important contributory factors to injuries on the slopes, that is fatigue, has received little attention outside academic circles. This may be due to the fact that all the major skiing manufacturers are either European or North American based and in these countries it is much more common to ski regularly at weekends, the ski fields being accessible to a greater proportion of the population. This means that people can take time to build up their levels of fitness without subjecting themselves to sudden, intense bouts of skiing. Also, with the frequent practice, they become technically better skiers more quickly, which in turn will offset the effects of fatigue. A more cynical explanation is, perhaps, that with no product to sell at the end of it the immediate and direct benefits of an organised ski fitness programme are not considered worthy of commercial investment.

What is needed is an effective and easily followed system of exercises which the average holiday skier can perform with the minimum of equipment. These should infringe as little as possible on the person's time, but offer definite progression over a series of weeks with the expressed target of, on a certain date, being Fit to Ski.

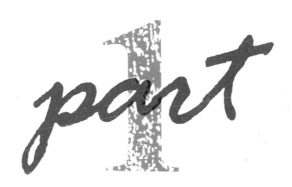

THE PROGRAMME

There are not very many ski fitness programmes around. Of those which do exist, none have managed to gain popular support, which in view of the enormous increase in the number of skiers seems to be somewhat odd. Why should this be so?

The most immediate answer is that they all suffer from being overwhelmingly boring, tending to be a tedious and directionless collection of exercises offering little encouragement to persevere. The average person who is going on a skiing holiday for only one or two weeks in the year is hardly going to be tempted to give up even a couple of hours in a busy weekly working schedule, irrespective of how sensible he or she knows it to be, to a haphazard collection of stretches and bends because someone somewhere says they are good for skiing but cannot be bothered to provide any guidelines beyond 'repeat ten times', and 'have a rest for a while'. What happens if I cannot do it ten times? How long do I rest for? What good am I doing anyway?

We cannot escape the fact that training for a sport by means of exercises is by its very nature boring. But it is not the actual choice of exercises that is the main cause of the unattractiveness of most ski programmes. Jane Fonda has, after all, made a fortune out of boring exercises. Her secret lay in the simple inclusion in her programme of three basic ingredients, namely music, company and a sense of purpose, all available within the structured framework of a class with well-informed instruction. People can see what they are trying to achieve, and why, and assess how near they are to achieving it. The result is that a set of consistently repetitive and unremarkable exercises succeeds in getting previously unathletic individuals up and moving and enjoying physical activity as never before.

These qualities of purpose and enjoyment are also offered by the Fit to Ski programme. It is undoubtedly more appealing if done to music (any music with a steady beat will do) and with other people. Your sense of purpose is firmly established by booking a skiing holiday, the date on which you have to be fit for skiing. The programme's structure enables progression in terms of difficulty and duration, and provides constant feedback as to how well you are performing. It is a programme as opposed to a collection of exercises, and I would strongly discourage you from simply picking out one or two exercises which specifically appeal and doing them at random, an approach which is for the most part quite useless. I would hope also that after reading the information set out in this book you will have a good idea of why each exercise has been chosen and what it is trying to achieve, as well as an appreciation of the overall goals.

In this way I would hope to persuade you, the busy working man or woman, that under two hours per week is a small and enjoyable price to pay for a more comfortable and infinitely more rewarding holiday.

Fitness for any sport is, to a certain extent, specific to that sport. An international athlete may be exceptionally fit and able at the one hundred metres, but a couple of lengths of a swimming pool may leave him breathless. This specificity of fitness is increasingly significant the more complicated the movements and skills for that sport become, and the more distanced they are from normal everyday activity. As skiing necessitates a complex series of movements and a broad and contrasting array of skills, most of which are not called for in such a way in any other activity or sport, it is essential that any ski fitness programme mimics as far as possible the kinds of stresses and strains you can expect to encounter on the slopes.

To this end, it is necessary to examine what aspects of fitness are required in skiing.

AEROBIC EFFICIENCY

All types of fitness are based on a bedrock of aerobic efficiency. This aspect of fitness deals with the transport of oxygen in the blood (aerobic means the presence of oxygen) from the lungs via the heart to the working tissues. It is this that provides us with endurance and stamina, which is what most people associate with fitness. A higher level of aerobic efficiency is what separates the tireless, forever active person from the individual for whom a short stroll to the local shops presents a major physical challenge. In skiing terms, it allows us to get through a day's skiing with greater ease and then on through the week more comfortably. Our capacity is largely determined by genetic factors (if you want to be an Olympic marathon runner, choose your parents!), but the ability to fulfil that genetic potential derives from training. With increasing aerobic fitness the inside of the heart becomes larger and allows it to pump more strongly, the muscles become increasingly efficient at removing oxygen from the blood and so develop a capacity to work harder for longer, new blood vessels grow into muscles commonly leading to a decrease in blood pressure in older individuals, and we need to rely less and less on the more tiring parts of our metabolism for energy (see below). It is in many ways the health related side of fitness.

To train for improvement in this type of fitness, we need to exercise at a steady, comfortable rate (around sixty to eighty-five percent maximum) constantly for between twenty to forty minutes, at least three times per week, although obviously beginners would have to build up to this level. It is the constancy of the exercise that matters. Examples of this type of training are jogging, cycling, swimming, exercise to music and rowing, and these are all useful supplements to the Fit to Ski programme.

One of the overall effects of the Fit to Ski programme will be an increase in aerobic efficiency.

ANAEROBIC CAPACITY

While it is essential to have a good baseline level of fitness, it is also necessary at frequent intervals and for relatively short periods of time to be able to increase the rate of energy expenditure markedly, to be able to step into a higher gear. This occurs, for instance, when skiing down a difficult slope or powering over a mogul field or simply when going fast. However, the aerobic part of our metabolism cannot produce energy at a fast enough rate to allow work at such high levels of intensity and so we have to acquire the fuel for this type of exercise from some other source. This is supplied by what is termed the anaerobic (literally, without oxygen) part of our metabolism. It is this which provides us with our physiological higher gear and enables us to increase our work rate quickly when necessary. If we suddenly run for a bus or rush up some stairs, it will be this which provides us with the energy to move. Unfortunately, a by-product of this anaerobic production of energy is a substance called lactic acid and the accumulation of this in the muscle will rapidly lead to fatigue, as anyone who has stood panting at a bus stop after a quick but unsuccessful dash will be aware. However, an efficient and well trained anaerobic system, that is, one with a greater capacity, will delay the onset of fatigue and reduce the time needed for recovery. It will thus enable us to ski at more physically challenging levels of intensity more frequently, as well as allowing us to catch the bus more often. Importantly, it will also decrease the degree and extent of any aching felt in the limbs and so allow progress at a faster but more comfortable rate.

This aspect of fitness is generally badly addressed in most ski fitness programmes. Either there is an inadequate emphasis placed upon it, ineffective exercises are performed or there is little or no progression allowed for.

In the Fit to Ski programme, both the individual block exercises and the bounding exercises as a group are designed to improve this particular part of our metabolism.

STRENGTH

As in every sport, strength is important in skiing. However, in many existing programmes it is frequently over-emphasised; there seems to be a blinkered belief that all that is required are set upon set of quadriceps (thigh muscle) exercises. The fact that the very young and very old ski perfectly well proves that strength 'per se' is not required to any marked degree. As with aerobic efficiency we do need an adequate baseline level on which to build the finer and less enduring aspects of ski fitness, but it is a nonsense to expect to be fit for skiing just because your legs are strong.

However, strength does have a place as part of a generalised ski fitness programme and in order to incorporate it effectively it is important to ensure that we are training the muscles that we are going to need in the way we are going to need them, rather than simply performing a variation of a normal weight training programme. Also, the exercises must be progressed in such a way as to allow adequate improvement. With these ideas in mind, we should now be able to dispense with probably the most universally practised skiing exercise, the wall-sit. This is the one in which you sit for as long as possible with your back

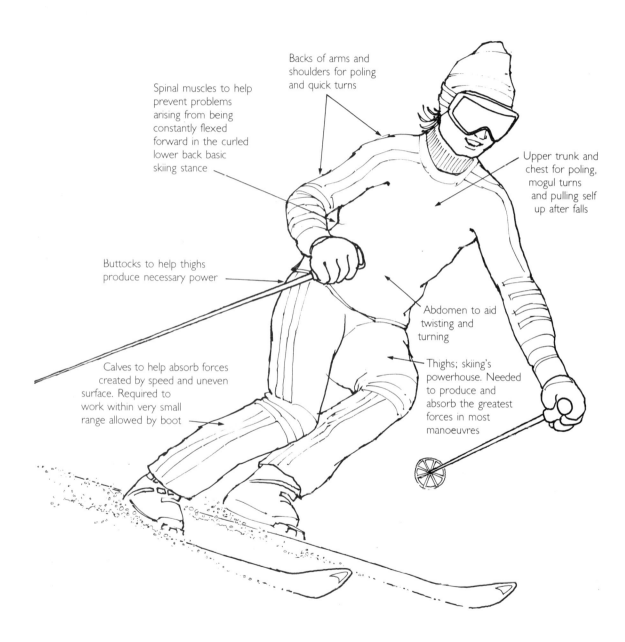

Backs of arms and
shoulders for poling
and quick turns

Spinal muscles to help
prevent problems
arising from being
constantly flexed
forward in the curled
lower back basic
skiing stance

Upper trunk and
chest for poling,
mogul turns
and pulling self
up after falls

Buttocks to help thighs
produce necessary power

Abdomen to aid
twisting and
turning

Calves to help absorb forces
created by speed and uneven
surface. Required to
work within very small
range allowed by boot

Thighs; skiing's
powerhouse. Needed
to produce and
absorb the greatest
forces in most
manoeuvres

against the wall and knees bent at 90° so that your thighs are parallel to the ground. It is supposed to build up strength in the thigh and mimic the stresses placed upon the muscles in skiing. It does neither. Moreover, two of the basic tenets of exercise prescription is that all exercises should be safe and effective. In my view, the wall-sit fails on both counts.

The back of the kneecap is covered with a special type of tissue called *articular hyaline cartilage*. This cartilage covers the articulating surfaces of most joints in the body. For healthy nutrition of this tissue alternate compression and relaxation is required and this is exactly what happens in skiing, the knees continuously flexing and extending as we adjust to the humps and bumps of the slope. If, however, we apply constant pressure, adequate nutrition will be hindered and possible damage may result; this is the case in the wall-sit. Also, it is an isometric exercise, that is, there is muscle contraction but no movement. Such exercise is associated with an increase in blood pressure when involving large muscle groups which can be hazardous in unfit or older people.

The effectiveness of the exercise is also highly questionable. Two of the principles of strength training are that the muscles should be exposed to a progressive overload and that they should be exercised throughout their range. Moreover, they should also mimic as closely as possible the activity they are trying to improve. The only load to which the wall-sit exposes muscles is your weight under the action of gravity. This is obviously a constant load and not progressed at all. The muscle is not stressed throughout its full range but just at a single point in its movement arc and any strength it does develop will be limited to that point. The exercise does not, therefore, adequately mimic what is required in skiing where there is constant movement at the hips, knees and ankles not a static contraction.

All the Fit to Ski exercises which involve an increase in resistance as the programme progresses are designed to improve strength. However, once a baseline level has been achieved, our aim is to maintain that level rather than work hard to increase it.

FLEXIBILITY

Flexibility is an important component of fitness for any sport. The human body is built for movement and action, but the comfortable, sedentary nature of many people's lifestyles today has meant that we have become a generally stiff population. This is especially true in the spine where postural problems resulting from decreased flexibility have led to headaches and back pain of near epidemic proportions.

However, it is commonly forgotten that not only is the *range* of our movements important, but also the *quality* of movement within that range. There is no point, for instance, in being able to touch your nose on your legs if to do so requires a three hour warm up and the forceful tugging of tissues as you creak and twist towards your goal! We need to be able to move freely and without resistance throughout all degrees of range otherwise any increase in movement we achieve through diligent stretching is for the most part completely wasted.

This is especially true in skiing where very little movement is actually performed at the end of range and apart from the smaller muscle of the calf (*soleus*), the ankle joint and the lower back, a high degree of flexibility is not required. What is certainly needed, however, is a fluency of movement, a smoothly flowing, efficiently produced series of motions like the well-oiled workings of a machine. We do not need, for the purposes of skiing, to work daily at stretching our knees and hips to their very extreme, we just need to be able to move them quickly and effortlessly through a normal degree of range. There is no necessity even to be able to touch your toes, but it is imperative to move within your limits with ease.

The warm up exercises in the Fit to Ski programme, therefore, have two main purposes: to ensure an adequate level of flexibility and then to produce and maintain a smooth and flowing movement within the range achieved.

BALANCE AND PROPRIOCEPTION

As we are skiing down a slope we are constantly bombarded with an incredible range of stimuli: heat, cold, brightness, speed, texture of snow, size of mogul and so on. Physical stimuli are picked up by specialised receptors in our joints, muscles and tendons which detect position, tension, speed and acceleration of different body parts. This is true for all types of activity whether it is as furious as skiing down a steep mogul run or as sedate as a walk through the countryside. The information gathered from this network of sensors is sent to the brain where it is processed and in response messages are sent down to the muscles to adapt to the new information being supplied. If on our country walk we suddenly trip over a branch or the ground becomes uneven, then this system enables us to take measures to correct ourselves immediately, measures which we presume to be automatic. Similarly, in skiing, if we unexpectedly hit a patch of ice on turning, the receptors will detect a sudden change in speed and acceleration and a probable slipping of position, and together with impulses coming in from our eyes which see the ice and our skin which feels the ice underfoot, this information will be sent to the brain which will respond by sending impulses to the muscles to lean the body further down the slope and cut the skis in more. This whole system of detection and response takes microseconds and is a continual process allowing us constantly to adapt to our environment. Our ability to respond to these mechanical stimuli is directly related to balance, and is termed *proprioception*.

While it is possible to have natural balance, it is not by any means entirely genetically determined and with correct training both balance and proprioception can be finely tuned and made more efficient. I believe that it is our ability to respond rapidly to changes in the position of our skis and body as dictated by our speed, direction and the nature of slope which above all else enables us to ski fluently and without injury. It is this central skill which separates expert from intermediate, intermediate from beginner. If, when walking, every time we turned a corner the necessary change in gait caused us to fall over, then simple motion would be an ungainly and uncomfortably slow process. So it is with skiing. If we do not know where our skis are without looking, if every time we go over a bump we fail to adapt our body position to compensate, if we face the wrong way up the slope at each turn, if every time one ski strays or catches in deep snow we do not readjust its position automatically, then skiing would be a maddening collection of tumbles and mounting frustrations. However, it is not possible to achieve these fluent adjustments if we are not strong, quick or fit enough to operate our responses effectively. In many ways a skier is like the female gymnast; she gets scored on grace and fluency of movement, yet without the strength or flexibility to complete the manoeuvres nor the anaerobic capacity to perform the routine nor the aerobic efficiency to compete all day and train all week, she cannot display the poise and balance for which she strives.

So balance and proprioception are the final objective of the 'Fit to Ski' skier. These are the eye-catching skills which will distinguish you from others and provide those special, breathtaking days when you manage to get it just right. Without a firm foundation of ski fitness on which to lay them, however, possessing these skills is an unfortunate waste of time and talent.

The exercises in the Fit to Ski programme which involve bounding and hopping followed by balancing and progressing to flexing the knees, hips and ankles with the eyes closed, are designed to aid and improve balance and proprioception.

DO ALL SKIERS NEED THE SAME LEVEL OF FITNESS?

The short answer to this is yes, if they all want to ski at the level of their capabilities. For instance, a beginner may have to pull on all his reserves of fitness to get down a simple green slope as he is skiing at the very edge of his ability, but an overweight and out of condition skiing instructor could probably cruise around all day on the same runs without ever getting breathless. The latter is obviously skiing well within himself and his technical ability masks his basic lack of fitness. If, however, he were to try to push himself to the extreme and attempt a difficult steep powder or fast downhill run, he would find his skiing technique progressively impaired by exhaustion, which would force him to stop one way or another!

Quite simply, if you wish to improve your skiing and so get more out of your holiday with every visit to the slopes, whether it is your first or twenty first outing you will need the same level of fitness. If you are content to cruise all day without even slightly taxing yourself, then you *may* get away with it. However, it is perhaps prudent to remember that the aches and pains of the three day blues are entirely due to fatigue and have served to dampen more skiing holidays than any sudden shower or thaw.

The programme itself is designed to last for five weeks with two sessions per week. Each session includes two different types of exercise, block exercises and bounding exercises. The time spent on each exercise is systematically increased each week, and both types of exercise are also progressed in terms of difficulty. The four groups of block exercises and four interspersed periods of bounding exercises are termed a 'circuit'. Two circuits are performed at each session.

Block exercises are the foundation exercises of the programme, the building blocks upon which it is structured. They are separate individual exercises designed to train different and specific parts of the body. They mainly result in an increase in anaerobic capacity and, to a lesser degree, strength.

Bounding exercises are different in that, unlike the block exercises, they are all similar to each other and are simply variations on a theme, the common aim being to improve the balance and proprioceptive systems, although anaerobic capacity will also be helped. These are the exercises which will help you acquire an immediate and certain knowledge of the position of each part of the body during the complex manoeuvres of skiing.

The overall effect of the programme will be an increase in aerobic efficiency.

THE BLOCK EXERCISES

Take a look at the chart on pages 22–23. There are sixteen block exercises and these are performed in groups of four. At the end of each group there is a period of bounding exercises before the next group begins. The performance times of, and the rest intervals in between, individual block exercises are of a specific length and are progressed over the five weeks as follows:

PROGRAMME CHART

PROGRESSION

	1	2	3
1 **Push Offs**			
2 **Hip Lifts**			
3 **Side Raises**			
4 **Cross Floor Jumps**			
Bounding Exercises			
5 **Shoulder backs**			
6 **Ankle Lifts**			
7 **Press ups**			
8 **Bucket Jumps**			
Bounding Exercises			
9 **Trunk lifts**			
10 **Sit ups**			
11 **Back raises**			
12 **Alternate squats**			
Bounding Exercises			
13 **Trunk rotations**			
14 **Stand ups**			
15 **Heel swings**			
16 **Forward & backward twists**			
Bounding Exercises			

Week 1 15s work 20s rest	Week 2 20s work 20s rest	Week 3 25s work 15s rest	Week 4 30s work 15s rest	Week 5 30s work 10s rest
1 min	1.25 min	1.5 min	2 mins	2.5 mins
1 min	1.25 min	1.5 min	2 mins	2.5 mins
1 min	1.25 min	1.5 min	2 mins	2.5 mins
1 min	1.25 min	1.5 min	2 mins	2.5 mins

	DURATION OF EXERCISE	REST INTERVAL
Week 1	15 seconds	20 seconds
Week 2	20 seconds	20 seconds
Week 3	25 seconds	15 seconds
Week 4	30 seconds	15 seconds
Week 5	30 seconds	10 seconds

The first session in the first week would therefore begin with fifteen seconds each of push offs, hip lifts, side raises and cross floor jumps, each with a twenty second rest interval in between, followed by the commencement of the first period of bounding exercises.

However, people differ widely in terms of strength and fitness and in order to accommodate this the first three exercises in each group can be performed at three levels, or progressions of difficulty. The easiest is progession 1, the most stressful, progression 3. It is up to you to decide at which level of difficulty to begin each exercise and also when to progress. Remember that strength and fitness also vary within different muscles of the body and if, for instance, you have strong arms but weak abdominal muscles you may wish to begin the push offs at progression 2 but the sit ups at progression 1. If there is any uncertainty, start at the easiest level. Please note also that men and women naturally differ in terms of strength of certain muscle groups. While this has no bearing on relative levels of fitness, it does mean that in trying to accommodate both sexes, the upper progressions of two of the exercises, press ups and side raises, will be beyond the natural physical capabilities of most women. This in no way detracts from the effectiveness of the programme for either men or women.

THE BOUNDING EXERCISES

After each group of four block exercises, bounding exercises are performed for a specified period. The duration of this period is again progressed throughout the weeks.

DURATION OF PERIOD OF BOUNDING EXERCISES	
Week 1	1 minute
Week 2	1.25 minutes
Week 3	1.5 minutes
Week 4	2 minutes
Week 5	2.5 minutes

STRUCTURE OF SESSION

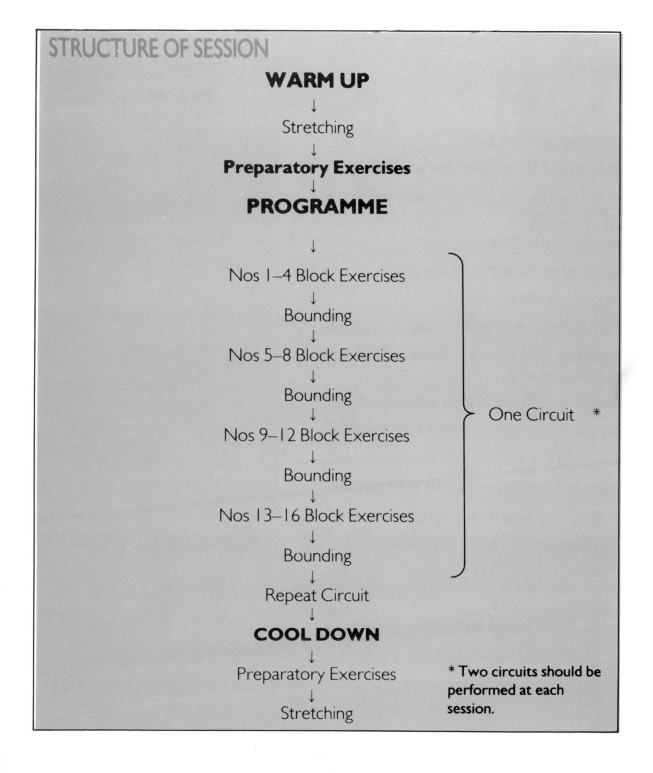

WARM UP
↓
Stretching
↓
Preparatory Exercises
↓
PROGRAMME
↓
Nos 1–4 Block Exercises
↓
Bounding
↓
Nos 5–8 Block Exercises
↓
Bounding
↓
Nos 9–12 Block Exercises
↓
Bounding
↓
Nos 13–16 Block Exercises
↓
Bounding

⎫
⎬ One Circuit *
⎭

↓
Repeat Circuit
↓
COOL DOWN
↓
Preparatory Exercises
↓
Stretching

* Two circuits should be performed at each session.

BOUNDING EXERCISES

Jumping side to side

Jumping side to side, forward & back

Jumping side to side, forward & back and diagonally

Striding side to side

Striding forward and back

Hopping side to side

Hopping side to side, forward & back

Hopping side to side, forward & back and diagonally

Jumping forwards and side to side

Jumping backwards and side to side

Hopping forwards and side to side

Hopping backwards and side to side

Leaping forwards onto one foot

Leaping backwards onto one foot

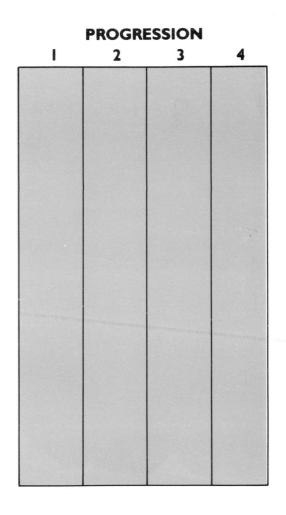

PROGRESSION

1	2	3	4

PROGRESSIONS

1 **Stopping and balancing on one leg**

2 **Stopping, bending knee to 45° and balancing**

3 **Stopping, bending knee, balancing, twisting twice to right and left**

5	Week 1 1 min	Week 2 1.25 min	Week 3 1.5 min	Week 4 2 min	Week 5 2.5 min

4 **Stopping, bending knee, balancing, twisting twice to right and left with eyes closed**

5 **Both bounding and balancing with eyes closed**

Look at the chart on page 26–27. You can see that there are fourteen bounding exercises in total and as it would obviously be impossible to cram all of these into each period, only a selection of them are performed each time. It does not matter which ones you choose or how many are performed in each period, as long as all are included in the session as a whole. Personally, I like to get at least four bounding exercises into each period, changing to a different exercise every fifteen to twenty-five seconds, but changing more or less often is just as effective. What matters most is continual effort; there should be no break between each exercise.

As with the block exercises, the bounding exercises are also progressed in terms of difficulty. There are five progressions in all and they are the same for each exercise. They involve interrupting the bounding with increasingly difficult periods of balancing.

The first progression involves halting the bounding at regular intervals and balancing on one leg; the second requires balancing on one leg with the knee slightly bent (around 45°); the third, balancing on one leg, knee slightly bent and twisting the upper body to look twice to the left and right; the fourth, balancing on one leg, knee slightly bent, twisting the upper body twice to the left and right with the eyes closed; the fifth, performing the majority of the exercises, including the bounding, with the eyes closed.

How many times to interrupt each exercise and how long to spend balancing is not a matter of precise timing. Mix them up. For instance, for the first period of the first week (you will be on progression 1) you may perform two bounding exercises in a minute, stopping four times for a few seconds to balance on one leg. For the second period, you may perform five bounding exercises in a minute, this time stopping twice to balance on one leg but for ten seconds at a time. Try all variations so that each session includes constantly changing periods of bounding and balancing. Again, remember that it is the unceasing quality of the exercise which is important.

Unlike the block exercises, everyone should start at progression one for the bounding exercises. Again, it is up to you to decide when to progress, but by the fourth week everyone should be up to the final progression and most of the bounding and balancing should be done with the eyes closed. This is not to say that the eyelids should be glued shut and allow you to become a stumbling wreck, a regular but swift peep to check everything is okay is all that is required to be able to teach the body to cope safely in the absence of visual stimuli. Obviously, all potentially dangerous objects which may be tripped over or bumped into should be removed from the room or rendered harmless, for instance, edges of carpets should be nailed down, anything on the floor should be cleared away.

WHEN SHOULD I BEGIN?

From the person who has remained inactive all year to someone who regularly participates in sports, the programme is designed to make everyone Fit to Ski within five weeks. The selection of progressions allows it to accommodate all levels of fitness and I would always recommend that the complete five week programme be followed. However, if someone is normally very active and can safely be declared fit, then it is possible for them to do only the last three weeks, that is, six sessions of the programme. It must be stressed, however, that this is the *minimum* level of participation. It is permissible to progress the duration of the exercises more swiftly if you feel you are not being stressed enough and, of course, the levels of difficulty can also be advanced, but at least six sessions are required by even the fittest athlete to allow the body to adapt to the unique physical and physiological stresses of skiing.

GENERAL GUIDELINES

1   Before starting on any exercise programme you should consult your doctor if you suffer from:

HIGH BLOOD PRESSURE
HIGH CHOLESTEROL LEVELS
ANY HEART PROBLEM
INFLAMED JOINTS

2   Care should be taken, and your doctor consulted in extreme cases if any of the following apply to you:

HEAVY SMOKER
HEAVY DRINKER
OVERWEIGHT
STRESSED
OVER 45
ON DRUGS
HAVE NOT EXERCISED FOR SOME TIME
PREDOMINANTLY SEDENTARY LIFESTYLE
INJURED JOINT(S) OR MUSCLE(S)
ANY OTHER PROBLEM WHICH MAY AFFECT YOUR HEALTH OR
ABILITY TO EXERCISE SAFELY

3   You should not feel *any* pain during the programme. If you do, then stop immediately.

4   The exercises are not meant to make you feel nauseous, dizzy or exhausted. If you do, then stop immediately, rest until symptoms have subsided for a while and begin again, but at the lowest progression in terms of difficulty and time. If the symptoms return, stop and consult your doctor at the next opportunity.

5   Work at your own pace. One of the advantages of doing exercises to time rather than performing a certain number of repetitions is that it enables you to adjust the exercise intensity

to your personal level of fitness. Be particularly aware of this if you are doing the programme with someone who is considerably fitter than you.

6   Do not exercise if you are feeling unwell, especially if you have or have had recently any viral-type of illness, for instance, the 'flu.

7   Do not exercise after a heavy meal. Allow at least three hours for digestion.

8   If you are pregnant, or think you might be, then consult your doctor before commencing the programme. If you are already doing the programme or are exercising regularly and you have no history of miscarriage and are feeling well, then there is no reason to stop exercising as long as you feel up to it.

9   The temperature of the room should be normal room temperature or slightly below, and well ventilated.

10   Wear comfortable, loose-fitting clothes. Wear extra layers if the room is cool and peel off as you warm up. Put any discarded clothes back on at the end of the session. Do not allow yourself to become cold.

11   Wear comfortable, well-padded, quality shoes, preferably with a thick sole, a stable heel and some form of ankle support. The present aerobic-type shoes are good.

12   The programme is more enjoyable if done to music and with other people, so get your friends round and party while you exercise.

13   The bounding part of the programme does tend to make a lot of noise, so make sure your neighbours are either informed, out or deaf!

Happy exercising!

Warming up

Before beginning any physical activity it is essential that you warm up. This increases the general temperature and mobility of the body which in turn increases the efficiency and activity of the muscles and, it is generally agreed, protects against stiffness and injury. There are many tales of people producing superlative performances without even so much as that perennial British favourite a roll of the hips and, indeed, firm scientific evidence for many of the supposed benefits of warming up is scarce. However, these stories are vastly outnumbered by accounts of torn muscles in cold athletes, and sprained joints in stiff ones. A brief look around any sports injury clinic on a Monday morning at the row upon row of otherwise fit-looking individuals bedecked to varying extents in tape and bandage, all looking regretful and murmuring 'if only . . .', should be enough to convince anyone of the necessity for a warm up.

However, the big problem with warming up is that even after having had its essential nature explained, the average skier, like most other sports people, simply does nothing. A few attempts at touching the toes and that ever popular but completely useless rotation of the hips is about as much controlled stretching as most skiers perform on holiday. Even when taking part in activities at home, most people shy away from correct warming up and content themselves with a quick jog on the spot and a roll of the shoulders.

The main reasons for this are boredom and laziness. Warm up exercises are boring and time-consuming, and people are lazy. It is understandably difficult when faced with a pristine slope and a brilliant day's skiing ahead to get down to the tedium of warming up rather than rushing straight off into the excitement of the day. Moreover, the first ski of the day is normally preceded by the now customary ordeal-by-transport — which can involve any number of different combinations of trains, buses, cars, bubble lifts, chair lifts, drag lifts and those ever-frustrating enemies of the holiday skier, queues. All this is suffered in anything from baking sunshine to freezing cold while you suffocate in your clothes and try vainly to master the art of walking with grace and efficiency with ski boots-cum-lead weights wedged on your feet! The only sure thing is that by the time you are ready to ski down the first slope, any warming up you have done back in your room will have, to a very large extent, been nullified. The best solution, therefore, is to provide a warm up routine which is as effective as possible in as short a time as possible, and is adaptable to whatever situation presents itself.

The Fit to Ski programme therefore includes two warm up regimes, one to be done before the performance of the programme, and a shortened version to be done before a day's skiing (from experience I think it is safe to presume that most people are even less likely to perform a lengthy programme in the less structured days of a holiday). The latter includes simple exercises designed to be performed in your ski gear when you emerge victorious at the top of the morning's first run. An effort has been made not to swamp the reader with exercises and neither regime purports to be *the* ideal warm up, but both are as short as a warm up for each particular situation can be without unnecessarily risking injury or hampering performance.

PROGRAMME WARM-UP – STAGE I
Stretching

Stretching is most effectively performed when the body has been generally warmed. It is, therefore, best to precede the stretching with two to five minutes of gentle constant exercise such as marching on the spot, slow jogging, cycling on a static bicycle or skipping.

Most people are acquainted with some form of stretching exercise even if it's just the automatic raised-arm-stretch-and-yawn on getting out of bed first thing in the morning. This natural impulse to stretch tissues which have lain in a shortened position all night and so become stiff neatly demonstrates your body's innate need for ease and fluency of movement.

The stretching exercises in the Fit to Ski programme are designed to ensure and maintain an adequate degree of flexibility and allow a free passage of movement.

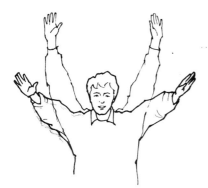

All the stretching movements must be performed smoothly and without jerking or bouncing. Apart from the first exercise, each stretch position should be held for five to six seconds and repeated four times unless otherwise stated. No pain should be experienced, just a gradual release of any tightness.

Backward arm circles

In standing position, circle arms smoothly backward in a wide arc for fifteen seconds.

Chin tuck

In standing position with hands on hips and keeping eyes and shoulders parallel to the ground, tuck chin in and turn head slowly to the right and hold for three seconds. Repeat other side.

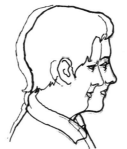

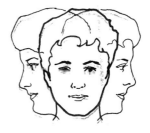

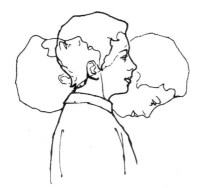

Neck stretch

Keeping shoulders parallel to the ground allow head slowly to fall back as far as is comfortable.† Hold for two seconds and bring head forward to rest chin as near as possible on chest.

Do not be tempted to roll neck in a circle as this grinds the small joints of the upper spine and may lead to damage.

† There is a misplaced notion amongst exercise specialists that extension (bending back) of the neck is inherently dangerous. Extension is a normal and essential movement, and lack of it in the lower cervical joints is one of the main causes of neck and shoulder pain, especially of the postural type. A rare number of people who suffer from certain conditions or anatomical anomalies may experience dizziness or "stars" in front of their eyes on bending their neck back, although this usually only occurs if the head is held back for too long or if the neck is also rotated. These individuals should return their head gently but immediately to the neutral position and not repeat the exercise.

Back rotation

Lie on back with arms and legs straight and arms approximately 70° to side, as shown. Keeping shoulders on floor, bend right knee slightly and bring right leg across body, attempting to touch left hand with right foot. Repeat other side.

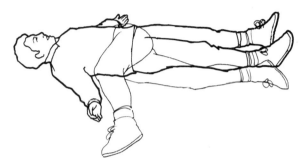

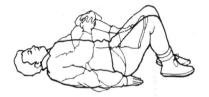

Back curl

Lie on your back with both knees bent. Keeping your head and shoulders on floor, hug knees to chest as shown.

Lean back

Lie on front with palms under shoulders, as shown. Push upper body up as far as possible without hips leaving floor.

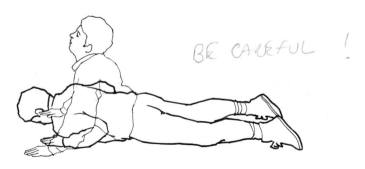

BE CAREFUL !

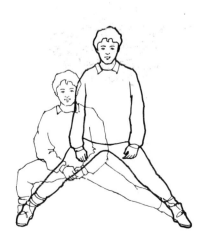

Mid-groin stretch

Stand with hands on hips, feet pointing forwards and legs as far apart as is comfortable. Bend right knee as far as possible without any part of either foot leaving floor. Repeat other side.

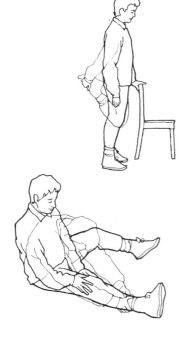

Again do not be tempted to roll or circle the hips as this does precious little other than to grind the joints of the lower back, and may lead to pain and possible damage.

Bent knee pull

Stand to right of chair with left hand resting on top. Keeping trunk erect, grasp right ankle with right hand behind you and pull right leg back as far is comfortable. Repeat other side.

Hamstring stretch

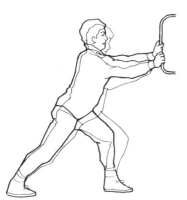

Sit with both legs apart with right leg straight and toes pointed and left leg slightly bent, as shown. Place both hands on right leg. Ensuring that the lower back is kept straight, bend forward at the hip, sliding hands down right leg as far as possible. Repeat other side.

Large calf stretch

Stand with left leg bent in front of you and right leg straight behind with both feet flat on floor, as shown. Keeping trunk erect, lean body forward as far as possible without right heel leaving floor. Repeat other side.

Small calf stretch

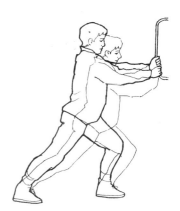

In above starting position, lean forward and bend left knee as far as possible without left heel leaving floor. Repeat other side.

PROGRAMME WARM-UP – STAGE 2

Preparatory exercises

These are designed to follow on from the stretching. They cause an increase in general body temperature, stimulating the circulation to tune the body's engine to an optimal working temperature, and mobilise the muscles and joints preparing them for the demands of exercise. They should be done in a smooth, rhythmical fashion and for fifteen seconds each.

Leg swings

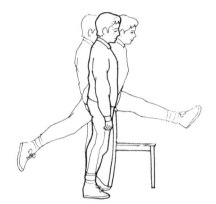

Stand to the right of a chair with left hand resting on top. Balancing on the left leg, swing right leg backwards and forwards as far as is comfortable, keeping knee straight but ankle relaxed. Repeat other side.

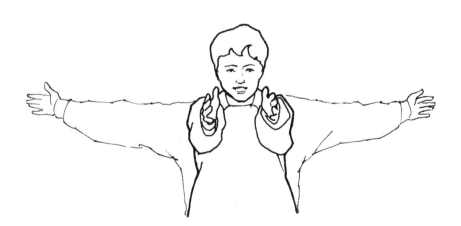

Horizontal arm swings

In standing position, keeping arms parallel to ground, swing arms forward and backwards and try to clap at the front and back.

Side leg raises

Lie on left side with left leg bent and right leg straight and head resting on the left hand, as shown. Keeping right leg straight and toes pointing forwards, raise right leg up and down in a controlled movement. Repeat other side.

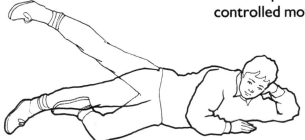

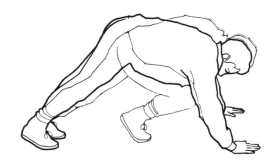

Alternate squat thrusts

Adopt press-up position where body is supported by hands and feet with elbows and knees straight, as shown. Keeping hands still, alternately jump right and left knees forward to elbows and back in a comfortable rhythm, ensuring that bottom is kept high and only minimal weight is placed through the knee in its forward bent position.

Jogging (fifteen seconds each)

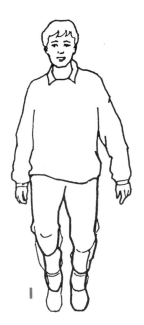

1 Jog on the spot, as shown left.

2 Jog on the spot, bringing knees up to level of hips.

3 Jog on spot, gently kicking heels in to bottom.

4 Jog on the spot, lifting knees as far out to the side as is comfortable.

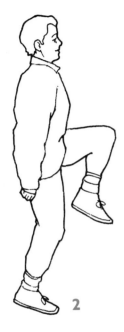

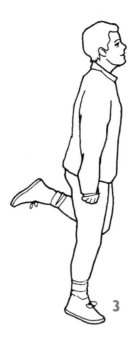

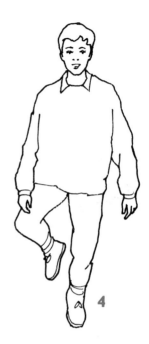

HOLIDAY WARM-UP

The unaccustomed physical stresses of skiing, the natural fatigue from exercising all day every day and the other less obvious but no less tiring rigours of the holiday – uncomfortable beds, late nights, duty free! – mean that your body normally wakes up aching and moaning to be left alone. This is when a decent warm up is most needed but, unfortunately, least often performed.

To make a positive attempt to help your body, use the following warm up regime. The first four exercises should be done in your room and the remaining five at the top of the first slope of the day, with your boots and ski clothes on but with your boots *undone*. Each stretch should be held for five seconds and repeated four times unless otherwise stated, and again, there should be no jerking or bouncing. Don't worry, you won't miss out on any breakfast or skiing, the whole lot should take no more than four to five minutes.

IN YOUR ROOM

Do the exercises as for Programme Warm-up – Stage 1.
Back rotation
Lean back
Bent knee pull
Small calf stretch

ON THE SLOPES

Back and leg stretch

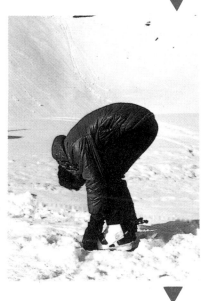

Bend forward with knees bent, hands touching toes and head tucked under so that chin is resting on or near to chest, as shown. Gradually straighten legs until you feel a comfortable stretch at the back of your thighs. Hold for five seconds. Slowly stand up, uncurling spine from the lower back upwards and sliding palms along the front of the legs. In standing position, place fists in the small of the lower back and bend backwards as far as is comfortable ensuring your knees do not bend and that your hips do not shift too far forward. Hold for four seconds. Reverse entire procedure and repeat twice more

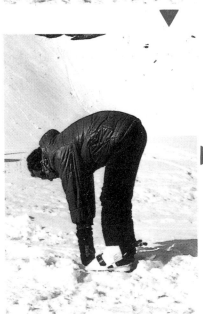
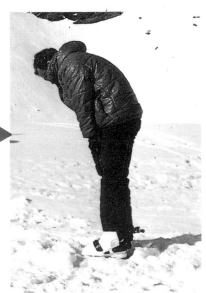
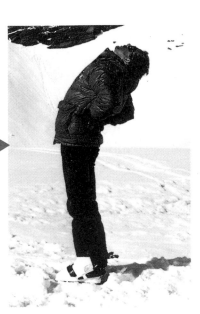

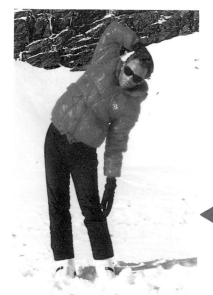

Side stretch

In standing position with legs apart, lay right arm over the top of your head so that the right palm is lying against left ear. Bend down to left as far as possible ensuring that upper body does not twist. Repeat other side.

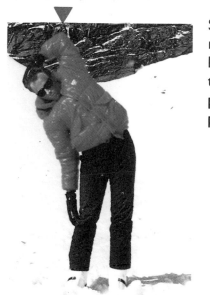

Trunk twists

Stand with legs together and poles in hands. In a controlled and rhythmical fashion, swing upper body round to the right, keeping pelvis level and lower half facing forwards, and touch the tips of the poles on the snow behind you as far round as possible. Perform six stretches on both sides and hold each position for two seconds only.

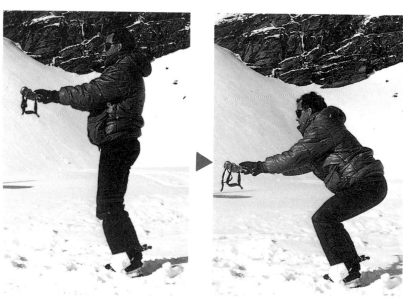

Half squats

In standing position, with poles held out in front of you as shown, bend knees to 90° and stand up again. Repeat ten times.

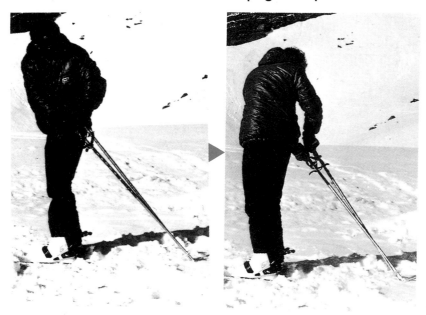

Each block exercise is illustrated with, where relevant, its progressions of difficulty and a description of which muscles and other parts of the body are being affected and their use in skiing.

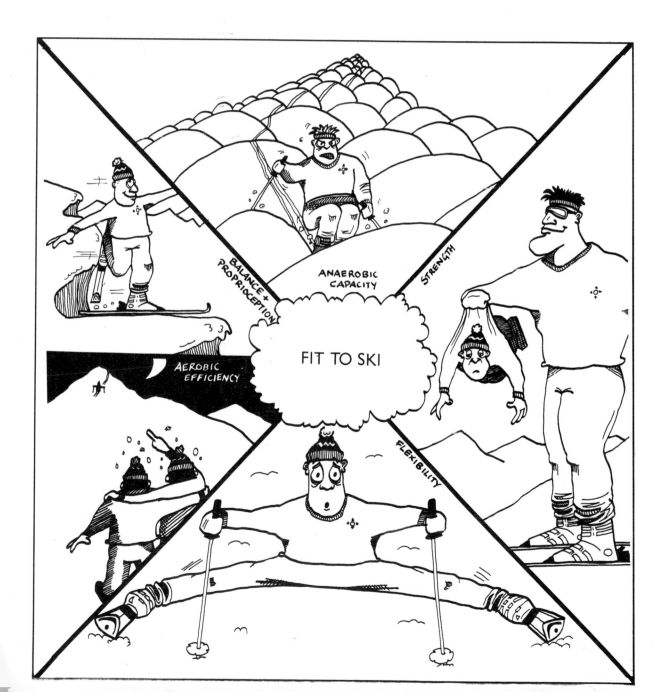

I PUSH OFFS

Progression I

Stand sideways on to wall with both your hands flat on the surface and elbows bent, as shown. Bend knees slightly but keep feet flat on floor.

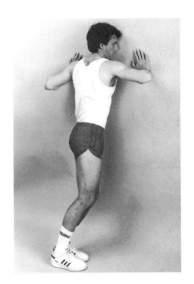

Progression 2

Adopt similar position as Progression I but with your hands flat on a chair and knees half bent as shown. If possible, the chair should be about knee height, or just below.

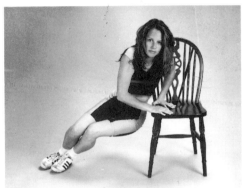

Progression 3

As progression 2, but return to sitting on each occasion.

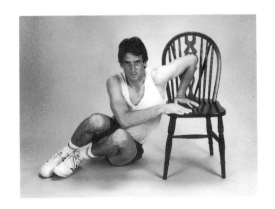

MUSCLES AFFECTED   Backs of arms; chest; buttocks; thighs

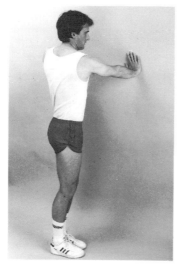

Push your body away from wall by straightening arms. Swap sides for second circuit.

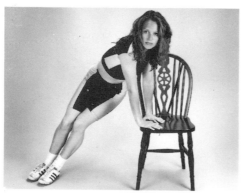

Push yourself into standing position by a combined straightening of the knees and elbows. Swap sides for second circuit.

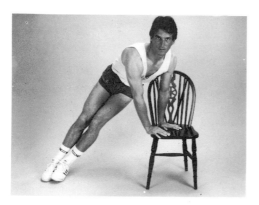

Swap sides for second circuit.

USES   Especially good for preparing for getting up and down from the ground on skis.

2 HIP LIFTS

Progression 1

Lie on your front with one
knee bent to 90°.

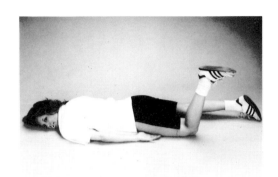

Progression 2

Lie on your back with both
knees bent and one ankle
resting on the other knee as
shown.

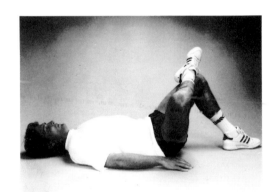

Progression 3

As Progression 2, but one leg
should be kept straight and not
allowed to touch the floor

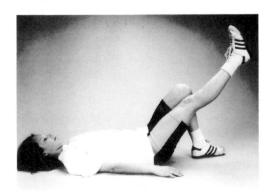

MUSCLES AFFECTED   Buttocks; thighs

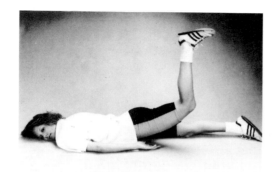

Lift knee off floor as far as possible. Swap legs for second circuit.

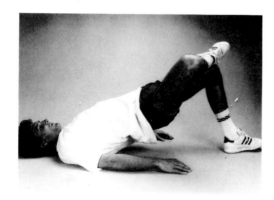

Lift buttocks as far as possible off the floor. Swap legs for second circuit.

Coaching Point *Avoid tendency to push down through arms*

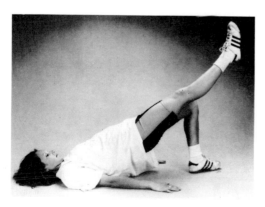

Coaching Point *Avoid tendency to push down through arms*

USES   Conditions lower limbs for general work of skiing.

3 SIDE RAISES

Progression 1

Stand straight with your hands on your head.

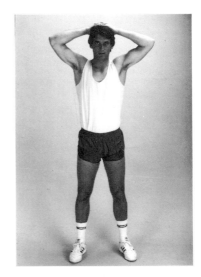

Progression 2

Lie on your side with lower arm wrapped around chest with elbow off the floor and upper arm resting along side.

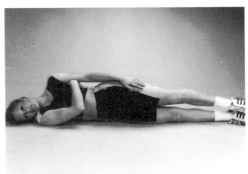

Progression 3

Lie on your side with your hands behind your head as shown.

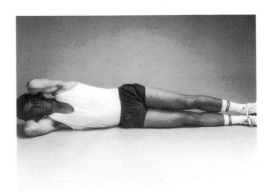

MUSCLES AFFECTED   The sides of the abdomen

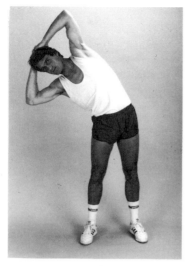

Bend to one side as far as possible and return to standing position. Swap sides for second circuit.

Coaching Point *Avoid leaning forward as you bend to the side*

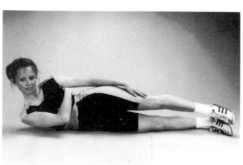

Try to slide upper arm as far as possible down side by lifting torso off the floor. Swap sides for second circuit.

Coaching Point *Avoid tendency to roll onto back as you lift up*

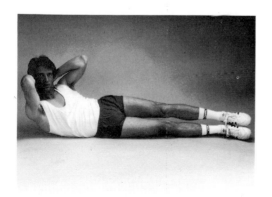

Lift upper body off floor. Swap sides for second circuit.

Coaching Point *Avoid tendency to roll onto back as you lift up*

USES   Needed for alternate side flexion involved in poling and quick parallel turns.

4 CROSS FLOOR JUMPS

Jump sideways back and forth across the floor as far and as quickly as possible, landing each time with your knees slightly bent and flexed inwards.

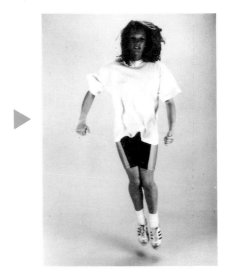

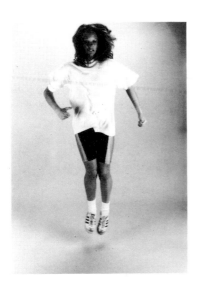

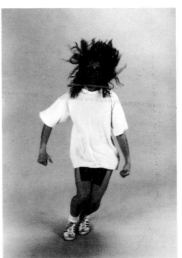

MUSCLES AFFECTED   Thighs; calfs; buttocks; good proprioceptive practice for knees especially

USES   Generally good anaerobic exercise which helps condition the thighs and calfs to the unnatural-feeling positions of skiing.

Bounding Exercises

FIRST OR FIFTH SESSION

5   SHOULDER BACKS

Progression   1

Lie on your front grasping a
broomstick behind you with
both hands.

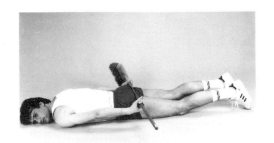

Progression   2

Sit on the floor with your
knees bent, leaning back
against wall with arms at 90° to
your trunk, as shown.

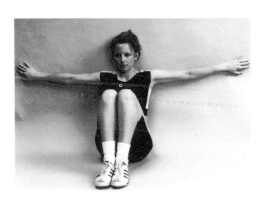

Progression   3

In standing position with your
knees straight, lean back
against wall with both arms at
90° to your body. Heels
should be about 12–18 inches
from the wall.

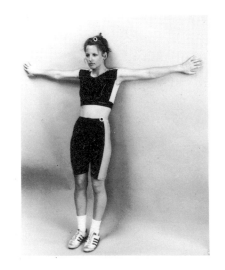

MUSCLES AFFECTED   The posterior parts of
the shoulders; upper back

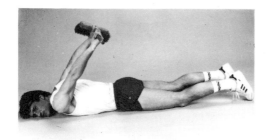

Keeping upper body on the floor, lift broomstick up and down as quickly as possible.

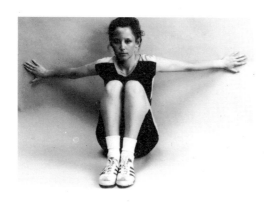

Push upper body forwards by pushing arms back in to wall.

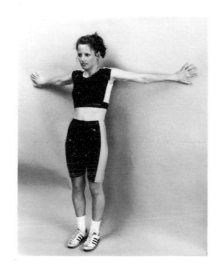

Push yourself away from wall by pushing arms back into wall, as shown.

USES Particularly useful for using the pole for extra power and on turning on a mogul.

6 ANKLE LIFTS

Progression 1

Stand with your knees bent at
approximately 45°.

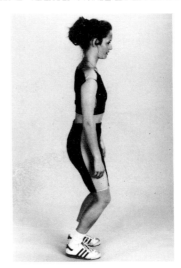

Progression 2

With your knees in the same
position as Progression 1,
jump up and down

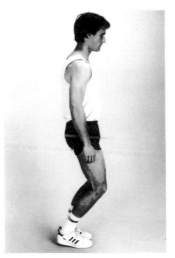

Progression 3

As Progression 2, but hopping
on one foot.

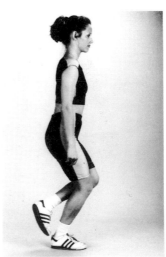

MUSCLES AFFECTED The smaller muscles of the
calfs; thighs

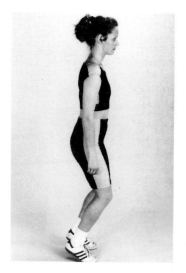

Raise body up and down on tip toes.

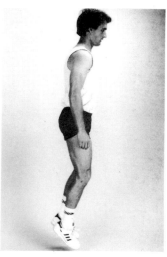

Coaching Point *Feet and heels should not slap down. If they do then calfs are too weak and/or movement is uncontrolled. Slow down, control movement or move to Progression 1.*

Swap legs for second circuit.

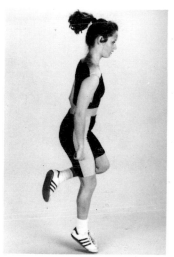

USES Prepares calf for unusual stress of physical activity while leaning forward, i.e. the position in ski boot.

7 PRESS UPS

Progression 1

Lean forwards against wall
with your elbows bent as
shown.

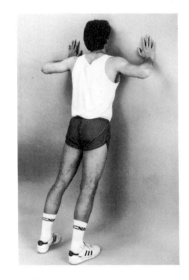

Progression 2

With your feet on the floor
and hands on a chair as shown.

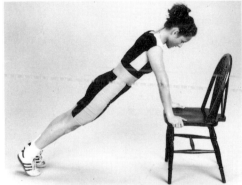

Progression 3

With your feet on a chair and
hands on floor.

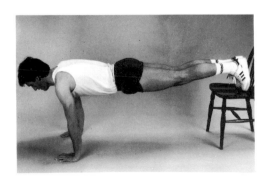

MUSCLES AFFECTED   Chest; backs of arms

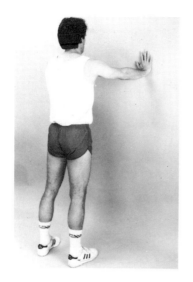

Push yourself away by straightening arms.

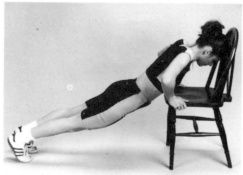

Lower chest to touch chair.

Coaching Point   *Keep back and legs straight, the tendency is to sag in the middle*

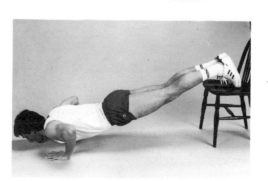

Lower chest to touch ground

Coaching Point   *Keep back and legs straight, the tendency is to sag in the middle*

USES   Poling and rising from ground using poles.

8 BUCKET JUMPS

Jump side to side over an upturned bucket as quickly as possible (if you are not entirely confident that you can clear the bucket with ease each time, then imagine a bucket rather than actually using one).

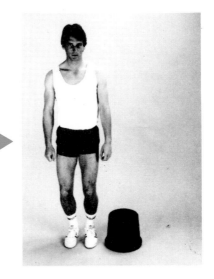

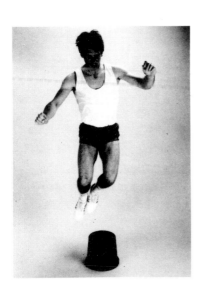

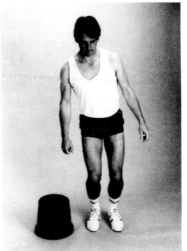

MUSCLES AFFECTED Thighs; calfs; buttocks; encourages natural "spring" in joints and other tissues

USES Excellent anaerobic and power exercise for legs. Physical preparation for the most difficult slopes.

Bounding Exercises

SECOND OR SIXTH SESSION

9 TRUNK LIFTS

Progression 1

Sit on a chair with your knees at 90°.

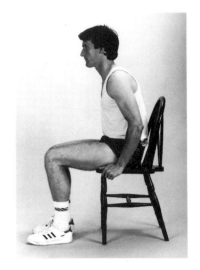

Progression 2

As Progression 1, but with your legs straight and only heels in contact with floor.

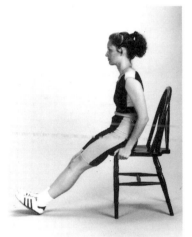

Progression 3

As progression 1, but with your feet not touching floor.

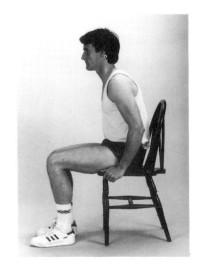

MUSCLES AFFECTED   Big trunk muscles at the upper back and sides; backs of arms

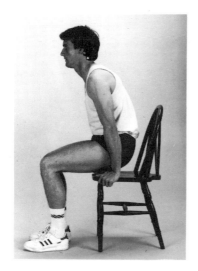

Keeping feet on floor, push through arms and lift trunk off the seat.

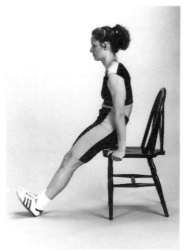

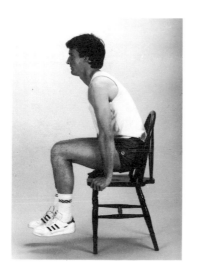

USES The major poling muscles.

10 SIT UPS

Progression 1

Lie with your arms by your side and knees bent.

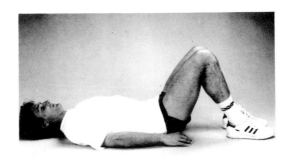

Progression 2

Lie as Progression 1 with your hands clasped behind your head.

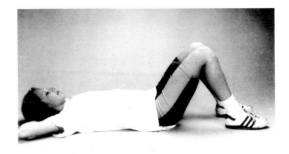

Progression 3

Lie as Progression 2 with one ankle resting on your opposite knee.

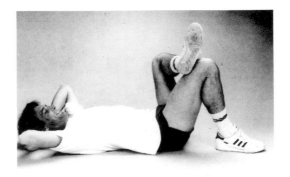

MUSCLES AFFECTED   The anterior muscles of the abdomen; the side muscles of the abdomen

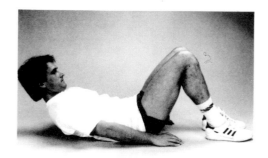

Keeping lower back in contact with ground, raise head and shoulders off the floor.

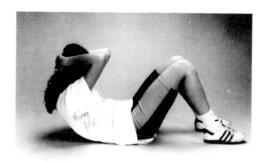

Raise trunk to an angle of approximately 40°, as shown. Lower back should be just off the floor.

Coaching Point *Avoid arching back and whipping body upwards. Control movement or go to Progression 1.*

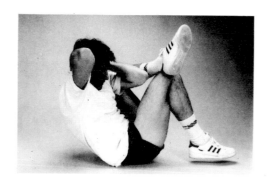

Bring elbow up to meet ankle of same side. Swap sides for second circuit.

USES   Provides the power for the twisting and turning of the upper body in skiing and also helps form a natural brace around the middle to protect from injury.

11   BACK RAISES

Progression   1

Lie on your front with arms by
your side and two pillows
under the abdomen, as shown
(your navel should be roughly
in the centre of the top pillow).

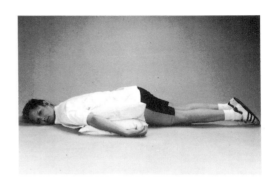

Progression   2

As Progression 1, but with
your hands resting on the sides
of the head, as shown.

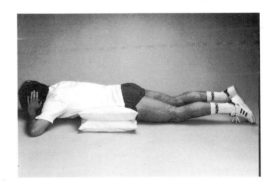

Progression   3

As Progression 1, but with
your arms stretched out in
front

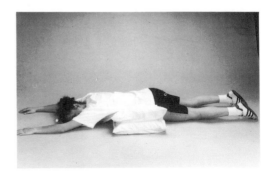

MUSCLES AFFECTED   Along the spine; back of trunk; buttocks

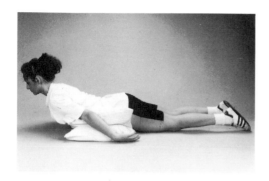

Lift upper body off floor.

Coaching Point *Ensure legs remain on floor as lifting trunk and lower body together can irritate parts of the lower back.*

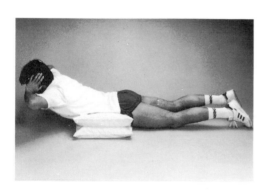

Coaching Point *Ensure legs remain on floor as lifting trunk and lower body together can irritate parts of the lower back.*

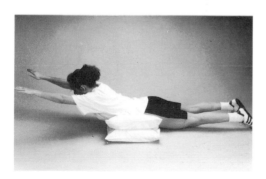

Coaching Point *Ensure legs remain on floor as lifting trunk and lower body together can irritate parts of the lower back.*

USES Provides resistance to the potentially damaging forces to the back which result from being constantly flexed forward in the curled lower back position of the basic skiing stance.

12 ALTERNATE SQUATS

Crouch with one leg in front
of the other, back erect and
fingers touching ground.
Jump, swap leg positions and
touch floor with fingers. Jump
and return to original position
as quickly as possible. Ensure
that legs are straightened
during each jump.

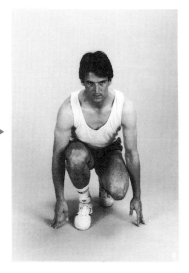

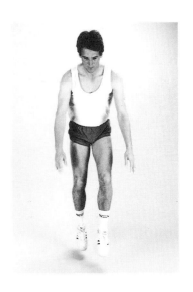

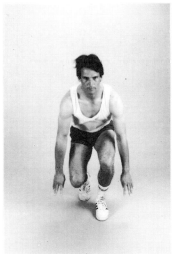

MUSCLES AFFECTED   Thighs; buttocks; calfs; encourages natural elastic spring of other
tissues

USES   Superb anaerobic exercise for the thighs. Mimics the hardest physical stresses
you will encounter.

Bounding Exercises

THIRD OR SEVENTH SESSION

13 TRUNK ROTATIONS

Progression 1

Lie on your back with your knees bent.

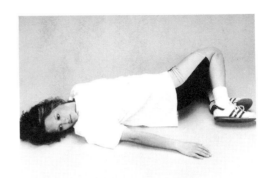

Progression 2

Lie on your back with feet off the floor and legs and hips bent at 90° as shown. Continue as Progression 1.

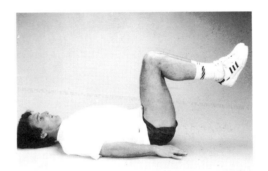

Progression 3

Lie on your back with knees and hips bent as shown. Continue as Progression 1.

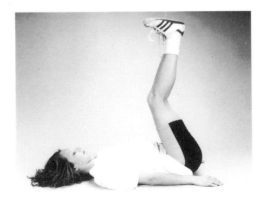

MUSCLES AFFECTED   Rotators of the trunk

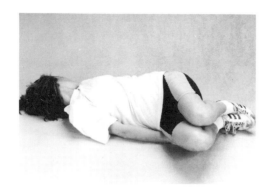

Rotate both knees to one side so they touch the floor and twist upper body the other way. Repeat other side.

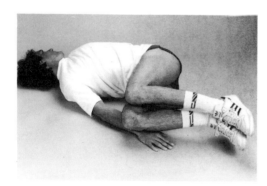

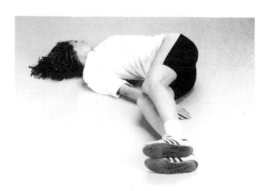

Coaching Point *Avoid temptation to push down through elbows.*

USES Helps twisting during turns.

14 STAND UPS

Progression 1

Stand facing some stairs. Step on to the second stair (third if you are very tall) and step down again.

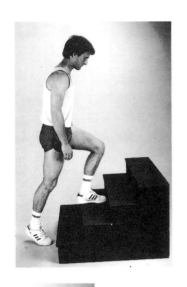

Progression 2

Sit with your bottom on the edge of a chair, knees bent at 90° and arms folded.

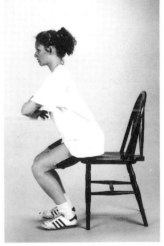

Progression 3

As Progression 2, but with one leg straight in front not touching ground.

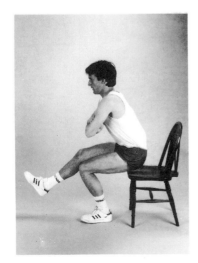

MUSCLES AFFECTED   Thighs; buttocks

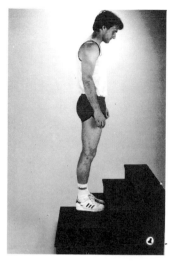

Begin movement with same leg up and down. Swap legs for next circuit.

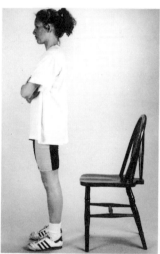

Stand up and sit down repeatedly, standing up again as soon as bottom touches chair.

Coaching Point   *Ensure that legs fully straighten each time you stand up*

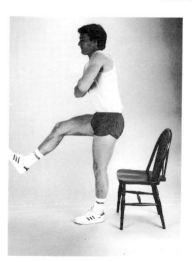

Coaching Point   *Ensure that legs fully straighten each time you stand up*

USES   Provides power and increases anaerobic capacity of skiing's powerhouse, the thighs.

15   HEEL SWINGS

Progression   1

Stand straight with your feet
rotated to one side.

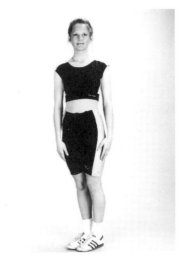

Progression   2

As Progression 1, but
alternately stand up on your
toes and rock back on heels.

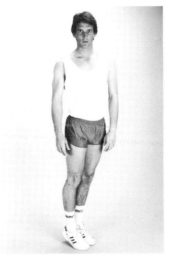

Progression   3

As Progression 2, but with
your knees bent to 45°.

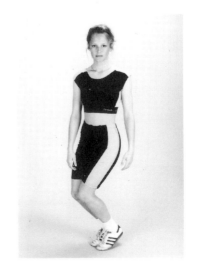

MUSCLES AFFECTED   Calfs; rotators of knee;
front of lower leg

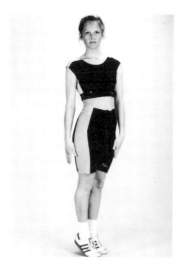

Raise yourself up on the toes, swing heels around and lower feet to ground. Walk both ways in this fashion.

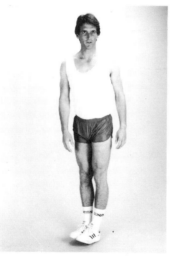

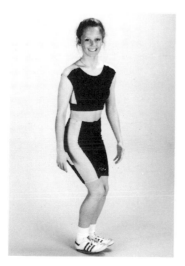

USES Helps to increase efficiency of proprioceptive reflexes in correcting unwanted rotation of skis.

16 FORWARD AND BACKWARD TWISTS

With your knees bent to 45°
jump forwards several times
and then backwards, twisting
hips and legs from side to side
but keeping your upper body
facing forwards.

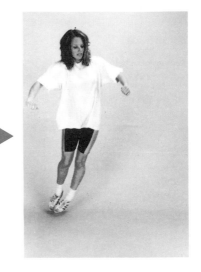

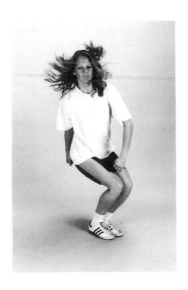

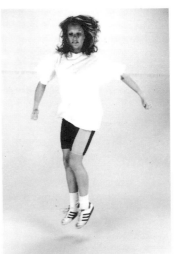

MUSCLES AFFECTED   Thighs; calfs; trunk rotators

USES   Excellent for training body to cope with physical activity within the
unorthodox pattern of movement demanded by skiing.

Bounding Exercises

FOURTH OR EIGHTH SESSION

The Bounding Exercises

To reiterate, the common aim of these exercises is to improve the balance and proprioceptive systems of the body and increase anaerobic capacity.

JUMPING SIDE TO SIDE . . .

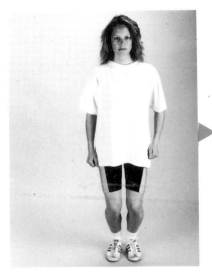 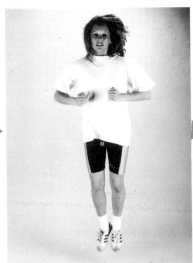 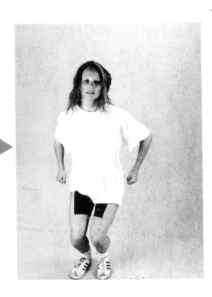

. . . FORWARD AND BACK

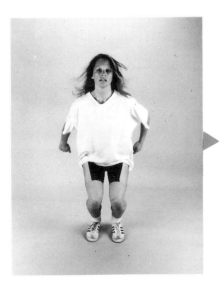 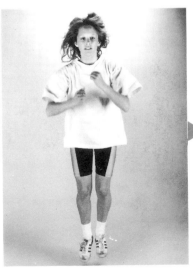 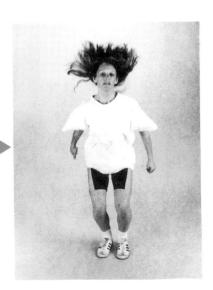

. . . FORWARD AND BACK, AND DIAGONALLY

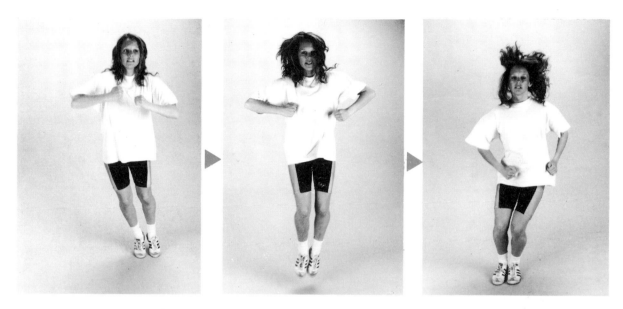

STRIDING SIDE TO SIDE

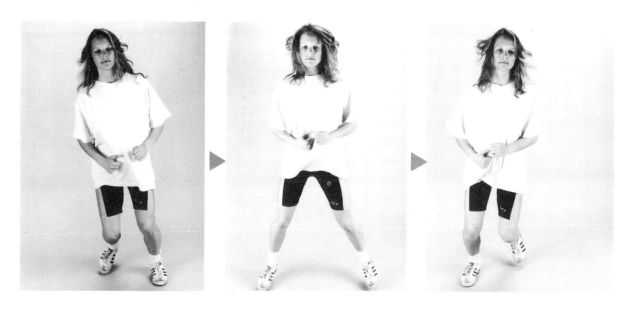

STRIDING FORWARD AND BACK

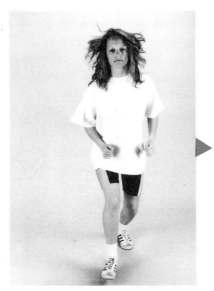 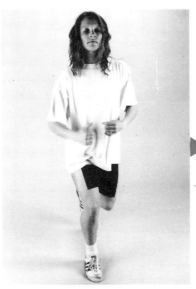 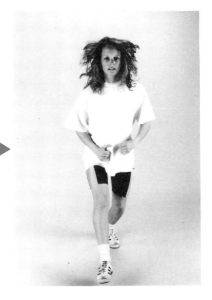

HOPPING SIDE TO SIDE . . .

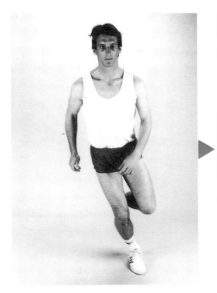 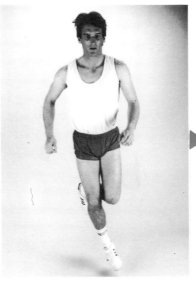 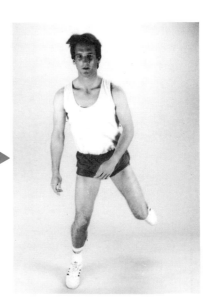

. . . FORWARD AND BACK

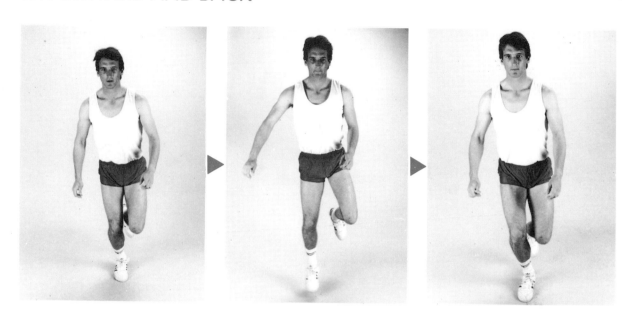

. . . FORWARD AND BACK, AND DIAGONALLY

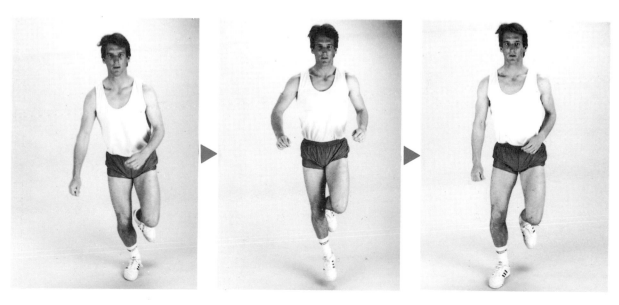

JUMPING FORWARDS AND SIDE TO SIDE

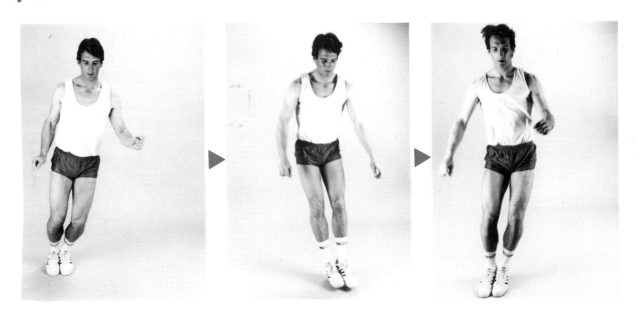

JUMPING BACKWARDS AND SIDE TO SIDE

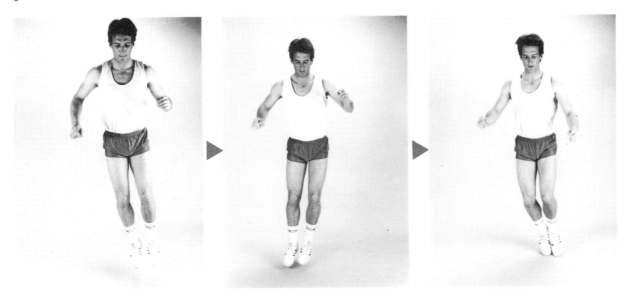

HOPPING FORWARDS AND SIDE TO SIDE

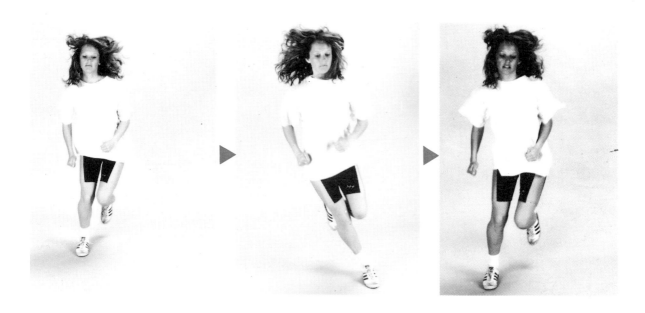

HOPPING BACKWARDS AND SIDE TO SIDE

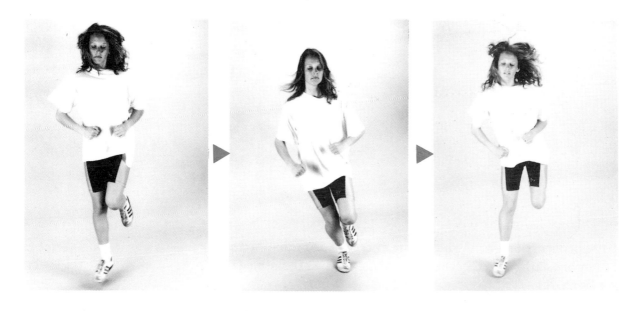

LEAPING FORWARDS ONTO ONE FOOT

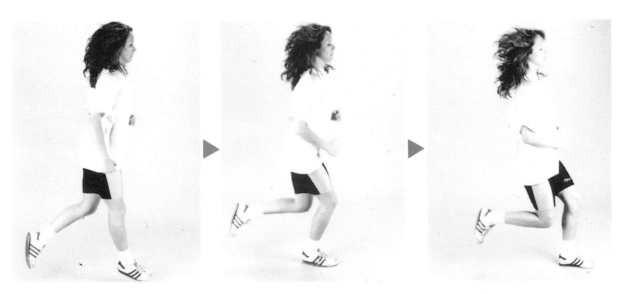

LEAPING BACKWARDS ONTO ONE FOOT

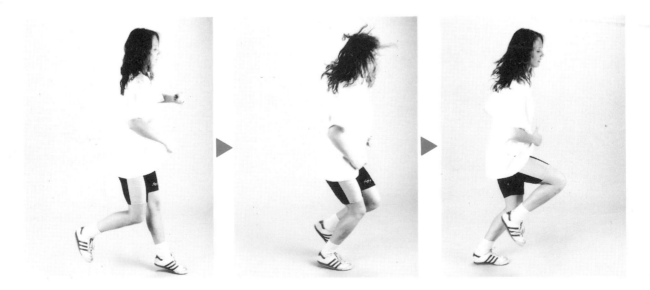

As the progressions for the bounding exercises are common to all, they are illustrated together after the exercises themselves have been described.

Progressions

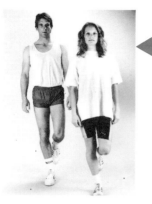

1   Stopping and balancing on one leg

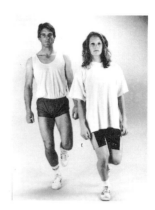

2   Stopping, bending knee to 45° and balancing

3   Stopping, bending knee, balancing, twisting twice to right and left

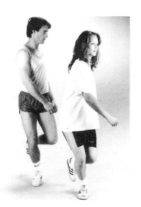 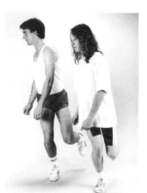

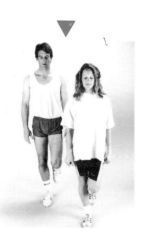 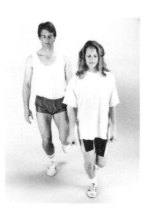 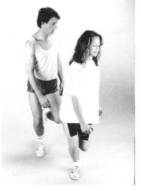 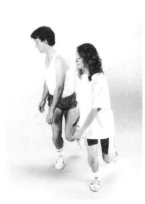

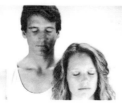

4   Stopping, bending knee, balancing, twisting twice to right and left with eyes closed

5 Both bounding and
balancing with eyes
closed

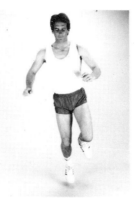

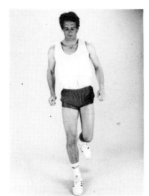

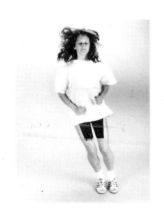

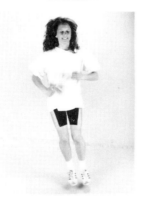

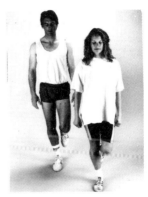

It is vital that at the end of a session of the Fit to Ski programme you do not suddenly stop exercising.

This can lead to a drop in blood pressure, fainting, and/or vomiting. It may also result in an increased risk of abnormal heartbeats and less seriously, although more commonly, an increase in post-exercise stiffness. Therefore, it is essential that you do not come to an abrupt halt, but gradually stop exercising or cool down. It does not matter how tired or pushed for time you are, if you simply slip on a sweatshirt and slump in an armchair, then you will not only feel considerably worse than if you had cooled down properly, but your heated and softened tissues will temporarily set in that position and on attempting to stand an hour or so later, you will find that you have mysteriously aged twenty years and that you creak and strain more than the chair you have been sitting on!

The best way to cool down is to repeat the warm-up, but in reverse order, so that the preparatory exercises come first followed by the stretching, with the difference that for the stretching exercises involving the legs – mid-groin stretch, bent knee pull, hamstring stretch, large and small calf stretch – each stretch position should be held for twelve seconds and repeated only twice. After that take a warm shower and relax.

On holiday, stretch when you get back to your accommodation by performing in reverse order the warm-up exercises done in your room in the morning. Make a concerted effort to do these, as they will help your body recover much more quickly from the strains of skiing and so allow you to ski more often and improve more swiftly. Considerable reward for a regime which takes as long as it does for your less diligent friends or chalet help to make the tea.

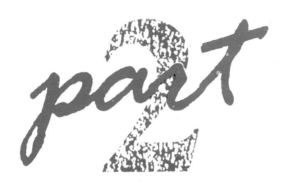

part 2

MANAGEMENT AND PREVENTION OF SKIING INJURIES

The tremendous surge in popularity which skiing has enjoyed in Britain over the past decade has been repeated, albeit less dramatically, throughout the developed world. There are now over fourteen million skiers in North America alone, ten million in Japan and in excess of thirty million in Europe.

The resulting increase in demands made on the skiing industry have had a marked effect on equipment, especially boots and bindings and piste preparation, with more money being spent on research and technical improvement. The overall result of this has been a quite startling decrease in the proportion of injuries, reported as a forty one percent drop over the last ten years. However, with so many people taking to skiing, there has been an inevitable increase in the number of reported skiing injuries. So much so that many experts now accept that these injuries constitute an international epidemic.

There are now around five million skiing injuries each year. Approximately one in twelve people will receive some sort of injury whilst skiing, around half of which will require medical attention, resulting in billions of pounds lost to industry and an incalculable cost in personal distress.

Why does skiing produce so many casualties? The reasons are varied but can generally be divided into those factors which we are able to influence and those which we cannot.

UNCONTROLLABLE FACTORS

Inherent dangers

Skiing has been said to be the most natural of sports: the skier is being powered solely by gravity. It is not like running where you can just stop if there are any problems. You are always being subjected to the influence of gravity and you must contend with this constantly to remain in control.

Hazardous terrain

With the increasing sophistication of modern ski resorts and their ability to offer every possible home comfort, it is easy to be fooled into thinking that the mountains have become a safe playground. But despite man's efforts they are still extremely wild and naturally filled with a great many potential dangers. These range from those which simply have to be avoided such as rocky outcrops, trees and avalanches, to those which have to be overcome and controlled, which may stretch from fresh powder to solid unyielding ice.

Climate

The climate in the mountains has the potential to injure and kill. At rapidly changing intervals it is subject to piercing sunlight, burning rays, freezing storms and mists so thick that it is literally impossible to tell the sky from the ground. You can get lost, frozen, burnt and blinded if you choose to ignore the basic rules of conduct and underestimate the climate's volatile and dangerous nature.

Other skiers

Anything from stray skis and poles to a straight collision with another skier is a distinct possibility on crowded slopes. Up to ten percent of all skiing accidents are as a result of collisions. Moreover 'second injury syndrome' is a not infrequent experience. This occurs after a skier has sustained an injury of some sort and is sitting or lying in the snow when another skier crashes into him or her, possibly causing far more serious injury, often to both parties.

CONTROLLABLE FACTORS

Fatigue

This has been shown time and time again to contribute to the likelihood of injury. Casualties often say that they felt extreme tiredness just before falling. As was discussed at the beginning of the book, people appear to think little of remaining relatively inactive all year and then suddenly exposing themselves daily to the physical demands of an arduous sport. Add to that the tendency to skip meals and the extravagant and liquid apres ski available nowadays and fatigue becomes a real problem. The third day blues is entirely due to fatigue and the aches and pains of unaccustomed activity. Most accidents occur around noon and between 3.30 and 5.00 p.m., that is, at the end of the morning and afternoon sessions when skiers are at their most tired. This has led to the development of the rule of threes – stop at 3.00 p.m. and go shopping on the third day and be careful above 3,000 m – which is sound but rarely followed advice for the ill-prepared. After all if you ski for only one week each year, whatever you are feeling you will still want to make full use of the time available and ski all day, every day.

The solution is twofold. Firstly and most importantly, follow the programme and get Fit to Ski. Secondly, ensure you are always adequately nourished.

Skiing is an energy sapping sport. Doing it all day and all week gradually depletes the muscles of the fuel they need for exercise and can lead to a creeping fatigue in even the fittest individuals, though the problem will be worse the more unfit you are. This fuel (called *glycogen*) derives from carbohydrates in our diet, and, as a car needs to be regularly filled with petrol, the body's engine similarly has to be frequently topped up with carbohydrate as energy stores become lowered. This is not to say that a brief visit to the nursery slopes requires six plates of spaghetti bolognese, but that regular meals and snacks should be eaten. The best foods to eat are those high in starch, such as bread, potatoes, pasta, cereals, muesli and rice, as these provide a long and continuous release of energy. Steer away from fatty foods. Fat is also used as a fuel (though not to the same extent), but most of us can be safe in the knowledge that we have enough of it stored away to see us through the lean times of a skiing holiday.† Make sure you don't miss breakfast;

† If you are spending prolonged periods living and working in very cold temperatures, then different dietary guidelines apply.

after a night's sleep the level of sugar in your blood will be lowered and it is this which regulates the distribution of energy to the muscles. If you have been drunk the night before, the problem will be compounded three-fold and a bowl of muesli and milk and a couple of slices of toast will be even more important, though infinitely less palatable! Don't skip lunch whilst on the slopes. It is important to replenish your energy stores after a morning's exertion, but be sensible, don't banquet on chips and beans as exercising on a full stomach creates its own dangers. A hot soup and some bread or a small pasta/rice dish will suffice. Also, take some fruit or muesli bars to eat during rest periods.

Fatigue is by far the most likely controllable factor which will expose you to injury and spoil your holiday.

Inexperience

It may be exhilarating whizzing uncontrollably down a black slope on your third day of skiing, but after one bad fall and a face full of snow, it may not only be your confidence which is irreparably broken. No one should tackle slopes and runs which they are not capable of handling safely. This is not taking the excitement out of skiing, it is taking a big slice of the danger out. Beginners account for fifty-eight percent of injuries, competent thirty-six percent and experts six percent. Apart from showing the importance of experience, it also shows that even if you are competent you are still six times more likely to get injured than an expert, which in view of the fact that experts tend to ski faster and in more potentially hazardous conditions, would tend to suggest that there are many skiers around the middle range who are not quite sure how average they really are. Peer pressure is one of the big problems. You must ignore it. Your friends may take great pleasure in showing you how easy a certain slope is and urging you to follow, but with five skiing holidays to your none their bravado is easily acquired. Know your own limitations and you will progress swiftly and safely.

Poor technique

Injuries to the knee, especially, are commonly as a result of poor technique (see page 105). Technique is best perfected with the aid of good tuition and practice. However, these are rarely available for long enough periods as anyone who, after a week of trying, finally masters a technique only to fly home the next day, will be all too frustratingly aware. We do not live in a country blessed with ski slopes accessible to the majority of the population and the opportunities to practise are therefore few. When we return to the slopes, maybe over a year later, we have to accept that, although a remarkable degree of ability will still be with us, we will not be able to ski immediately at the level achieved on the previous holiday. Those initial few days are the most dangerous, so beware.

If you do find your technique is constantly letting you down and especially if you cannot work out why, then get some expert advice. Skiing is an expensive holiday, it is pointless spending it in a maddening succession of falls. As well as feeling bruised and aching, you will become tense and anxious which will only serve to make your technique worse. Get some lessons. After all, the price of a round of drinks in most French and Swiss ski resorts should cover it!

As with all sports, however, some people will naturally and swiftly pick up the complex techniques necessary to ski well and others, despite good tuition, diligence and application, will never quite get there. This has to be accepted, especially if you fall into the latter category. Again, know your own limitations.

Speed

Going too fast, especially when linked with the above three factors, should pretty well guarantee a tumble. You are quite simply not as in control as you should be and are increasing not only the likelihood, but also the possible severity of injury. You must ski at your own pace. This is admittedly hard when you are skiing in a group, all of whom are budding Olympic downhillers and who are constantly having to wait for you. Let them go on or let them wait, it's your holiday too! If it is becoming a real problem try to find someone who is willing to ski at your pace. There is not much of a choice between skiing alone and skiing out of control.

Equipment

The progress in skiing equipment safety has been quite remarkable over the last ten years and, as was mentioned earlier, has been largely responsible for the dramatic reduction in skiing accident rates. However, too often the benefits of safer equipment are lost due to incorrect use and poor care and maintenance. For example, twenty percent of safety bindings are not properly adjusted and various studies have indicated that between sixty-four percent and eighty-four percent of lower-leg injuries could be prevented by correct binding settings. It is obvious that many skiing casualties could be avoided if everyone followed simple guidelines on the checking and use of their equipment.

Before beginning the day's skiing, everyone should check that their bindings are operating correctly. It only takes a minute or so and may save you from an abrupt and painful end to your holiday, and months of regret.

To ensure the toe release is working properly, stand with one ski on and kick the front of the boot with the heel of the other boot. It should only take a gentle kick to release the bindings. To check the heel release, again stand with one ski on and step forward with the other foot. The heel of the boot should lift out of the bindings. Repeat these checks after any fall which may affect the tension adjustments and regularly note the indicated release settings.

In many European resorts the tendency is to set the heel too tightly. If this is the case, or if the toe release is also giving cause for concern, then get the bindings loosened. Only tighten the bindings if the ski prematurely releases or if you are an experienced racer.

If the skis are your own, ensure that they are properly maintained and that you routinely lubricate all surfaces of the binding with a thin film of silicone to prevent icing and corrosion. Everyone should check their equipment for wear

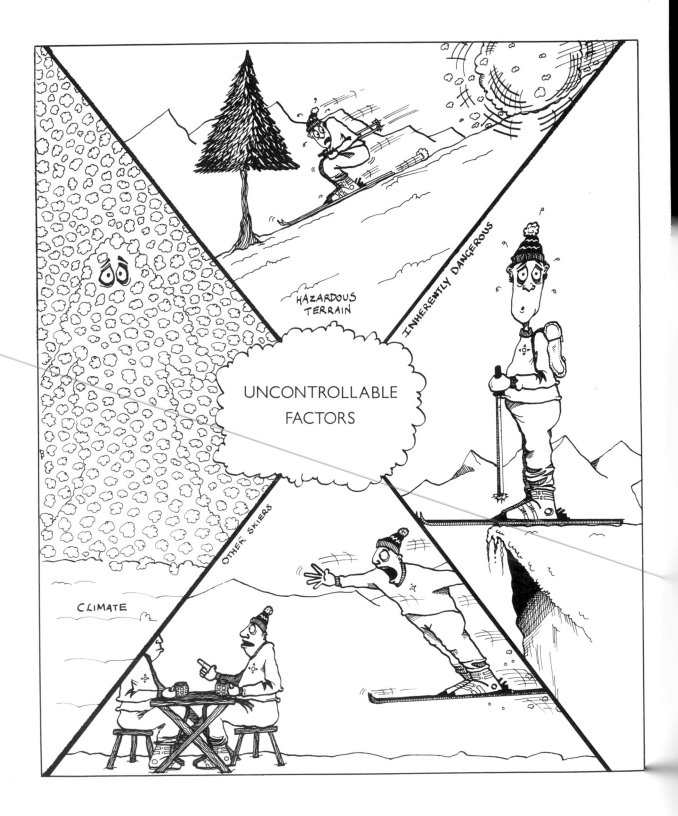

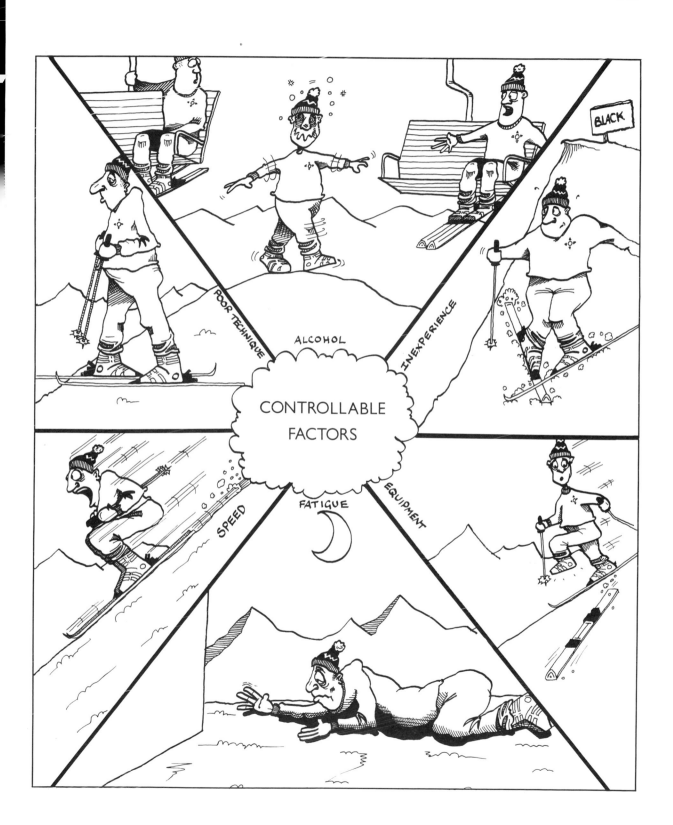

and damage, especially after a fall or skiing on worn pistes. If your skis are rented and you are not entirely happy with them, then take them back. They are charging you enough for them, so don't break a leg on their account. If conditions are icy you may want your edges sharpened. This takes very little time so do not think you are inconveniencing anyone, even if the assistant may intimate otherwise.

Make sure your boots fit correctly and that the insoles are dry. If you are buying new ski boots, buy them at least a month before you go and wear them around the house to break them in. Avoid walking on hard gravely surfaces with ski boots on as this may damage the surfaces which mate with the bindings. Always clean the boot sole of ice, snow and dirt before putting skis on.

Ski poles are particularly associated with thumb injuries (see p.98) so make sure you grip the pole outside the strap (p.99) to lessen the chances of the pole pushing the thumb backwards.

Do make an effort to follow these guidelines. To ignore them or to claim lack of time is simply to deny yourself the benefits of the excellent equipment available nowadays and to risk unnecessary injury.

Alcohol

Alcohol dulls the senses, inhibits judgement, disturbs coordination and encourages risk taking behaviour. It also makes you more susceptible to hypothermia, a fact which may seem particularly pertinent when you lie injured at the bottom of a black slope down which you have just attempted to snow-plough, inspired by an idea that seemed quite sensible at the time. In Austria, studies have shown that alcohol is a significant factor in up to a quarter of all patients hospitalised as a result of skiing accidents. So don't be stupid, don't drink at all on the mountains. Leave the glühweins till the end of the day when the journey home isn't so far.

GENERAL GUIDELINES ON THE USE OF STRAPPING AND ICE PACKS

Strapping

Some simple strapping techniques are described in the management of several of the following injuries. In all cases it is important that before the strapping is applied the skin should be clean, dry, undamaged and shaven. Please do not ignore the last point, even though the agony of tugging out each individual hair follicle as the tape is removed is a purgatory which every macho sportsman appears to have to go through before vanity can be replaced by common sense. It is a mistake even the bravest of the brave make only once.

The strapping should be applied firmly but not so tightly as to impinge upon the circulation. If there is any colour change in the skin, pins and needles, pain, numbness or irritation of the skin, then the strapping should be removed immediately.

Unless otherwise stated, the best strapping to use is porous elastic adhesive bandage, the most readily available brands in Britain being *Elastoplast* and *Leukoband* (7.5 cms width is the most useful size); these can be bought from most large chemists. In the case of the thumb (page 99) the more rigid, non-elastic 'zinc oxide' tape 3.75 cms width should be used. This can be bought from the same outlets.

Ice packs

When ice packs are used in the management of injuries it is of vital importance that the ice is not directly applied to the skin but first wrapped in a wet towel. Crushed ice is the best to use as this will mould more easily and effectively around the part being treated, but ordinary ice cubes and even a packet of frozen peas can also be used. If the part to be treated has for any reason a lack of normal sensation, perhaps due to past injury or frostbite, or if there are any circulatory problems, then ice packs should not be used.

Injuries to the upper limb account for twenty-five percent of all ski injuries and eighteen percent of the most common. While less frequent than lower limb injuries, they are undergoing a relative increase in number. The major reason for this is that the marked technical improvements in boots, bindings and skis have not been successfully repeated in the pole despite a variety of innovations, and the ski pole remains a significant contributory factor to injuries to the upper limb.

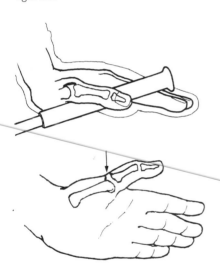

In a forward fall, pole pushes thumb outwards and backwards injuring ligament.

THUMB

Injuries to the thumb make up ten to eighteen percent of all skiing injuries.

The vast majority of injuries to the thumb involve the ligament at the base of the inside of the thumb (the *ulnar collateral ligament)*. It is usually badly sprained or ruptured and is known as game-keeper's thumb (so called because game-keepers would commonly injure this ligament on breaking their prey's neck!). There may also be an accompanying fracture.

These injuries are very much affected by the pole. They usually occur when the skier falls forward and naturally thrusts his or her arm out to cushion the anticipated impact. As is usually the case, the ski pole is still in the hand and the usual grip forces the thumb backwards and outwards. When the pole makes contact with the snow it acts as a lever and this gripping position is pushed to the extreme causing the ligament to rupture.

Signs

Pain, especially when the thumb is moved sidewards away from the palm; localised tenderness around the inside of the base of the thumb; swelling; painful weakness of grip; feeling of instability.

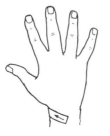

Hold hand palm downwards. Relax thumb. Begin centre back of wrist . . .

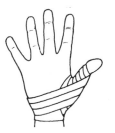

draw tape forward around base of thumb, turning hand as you do so. Bring tape up through between thumb and finger, then down around base.

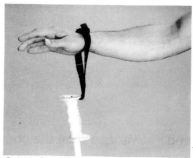

Continue across palm, applying tension through tap, and around back of wrist. Repeat 3 times until injured joint is covered.

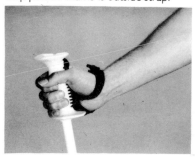

Grip pole so thumb is outside strap.

Management

If it is only a sprain, apply an ice pack for up to ten minutes at a time at frequent intervals for the first forty-eight hours and compress firmly with a strapping or bandage. When skiing, strap in such a way as to inhibit extreme backward and outward movement of the thumb (see left: for this strapping, the more rigid, non-elastic, zinc oxide tape should be used). Begin gentle gripping exercises after twenty-four hours.

If there is considerable swelling and pain and the thumb feels weak, then the injury is more serious and medical opinion should be sought as surgery is often necessary to repair the ligament and this needs to be done as soon as possible.

These injuries are often under-reported or overlooked so if in doubt, always suspect the worst and consult a doctor.

Prevention

It has been found that what matters is not the type of grip on the pole, despite this being the area where much equipment-related research has been concentrated, but the ability to get rid of the pole during a fall. Therefore, it is best to grip the pole outside the strap as this would make getting rid of the pole easier.

This injury is also very common on dry ski-slopes and occurs when the skier falls over and catches a thumb in one of the holes in the surface. It is advisable, therefore, when skiing on a dry slope, that a glove with webbing between the thumb and index finger which would prevent the injurious movement be worn. These gloves have been tried on snow slopes, but have often been discarded as being too cumbersome and restrictive. However, it is worth persevering with them as a bad injury to the thumb can lead to considerable disability and many weeks off work.

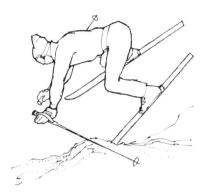

Skier falls forward, pole pushes arm up, back and around. Shoulder dislocates.

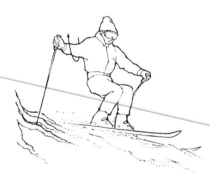

Pole catches in roots of tree. Arm is forcibly pulled back. Shoulder dislocates.

SHOULDER DISLOCATIONS

Two to six percent of skiing injuries involve dislocation of the shoulder. There are three main mechanisms of dislocation, two of them, again, involving the pole. Either the ski pole basket catches on a stationary object such as the roots of a tree and pulls the arm forcibly back, or the skier falls forward and the pole pushes the arm up, back and around. The third mechanism occurs when the skier falls directly on to the shoulder. The latter is more common in hard or icy conditions.

Signs

Intense pain; rapid swelling; the shoulder looks deformed; there is a gap where the top of the arm should be and a visible bulge where it now rests under the *clavicle* (collar-bone); the arm may appear slightly longer; there will be considerable spasm with all the surrounding muscles tightly contracting and prominent; the patient will resist any motion.

Management

Do not try to reduce the dislocation (put the shoulder back in). You are more likely to cause further damage. The only thing to do is to place the arm in a sling – a collar and cuff type is the simplest and best and can be made easily from an scarf (see page 101) – and go to a doctor. If the shoulder reduces spontaneously, medical opinion is still imperative.

Prevention

The shoulder is a naturally loose joint. This allows a great range of movement but does leave it prone to dislocation. Its stability is provided almost completely by the surrounding muscles and the most effective way of preventing shoulder dislocations is to build up the strength of these muscles and their ability to react to sudden stress through their entire range.

However, even the strongest shoulder will dislocate under the right conditions, so it pays to be aware of any objects

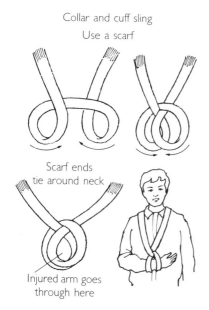

Collar and cuff sling
Use a scarf

Scarf ends
tie around neck

Injured arm goes
through here

under or around the surface which the ski pole may catch, especially when skiing through wooded terrain where branches, trunks and roots can all present hidden hazards. Some skiers, particularly in Canada, actually take their hands right out of the straps so they can let the ski pole go completely before any damage is done.

If falling forwards, I always try to bend my elbows slightly and turn my wrists inwards so that the back of my hand is uppermost as this leaves the shoulder less prone to dislocation. However, you need to have a certain degree of strength to be able to cushion the fall in this position and, remember, it is a natural instinct you are trying to overcome and you will not be able to do this immediately. Some people suggest that this action makes wrist injuries more likely, but I have not found this to be the case.

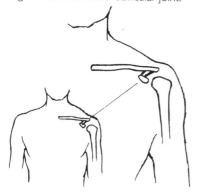

A fall directly on point of shoulder commonly injures acromio-clavicular joint.

Ligaments of acromio-clavicular joint.

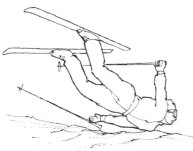

ACROMIO-CLAVICULAR JOINT

The *acromio-clavicular joint* is the joint which connects the clavicle with the shoulder (the point of attachment being the *acromion process*). Injury to it involves sprain or rupture of one or both of the two ligaments which hold the clavicle in place. This almost exclusively occurs when the skier falls directly on the point of the shoulder. Hard ice and high speed increase the chances of this injury.

Signs

If mild – localised tenderness; localised swelling; able to move the arm through full range without an increase in pain.

If severe – increased pain radiating from shoulder to neck; increased, but still localised swelling; unable to lift arm without pain; obvious 'step' deformity where the end of the clavicle has slipped upwards.

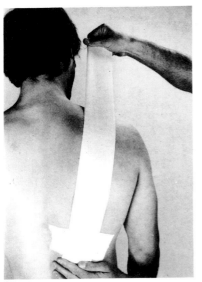

Acromio-clavicular joint is identified by 2mm crevice between collar bone and shoulder (see arrow below). Fix two pieces of strapping tape about 6ins long to back and chest as shown.

From 2ins below tape on back, draw a long length of strapping up over shoulder passing just to inside of painful joint. Applying downward pressure, fix to just below tape on chest. Lock ends with two small pieces of tape (not shown).

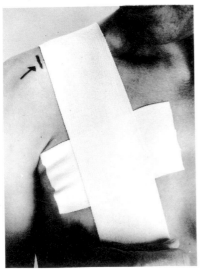

Management

If injury is mild, treat with ice packs for up to ten minutes as and when necessary and continue for the whole skiing trip. Place in a sling for comfort. The condition is self-limiting and if the pain is not bad enough to prevent you from skiing, then no further harm will be done to the joint by doing so. Strapping applied as shown left will probably help.

If the injury is severe, again medical opinion must be sought as untreated acromio-clavicular injuries commonly cause residual symptoms. Surgery is a possibility but not strictly necessary even in the most severe injuries. Splinting or simply rest may be advised according to prevailing orthopaedic opinion.

Prevention

As the acromio-clavicular joint is not under the direct control of any muscle groups, specific strengthening exercises will not prevent injury (they may, however, be necessary after injury occurs and wasting of the surrounding musculature ensues). However, as the injury almost exclusively happen in falls and especially when skiing fast in icy conditions, the need for skiing within your own limitations and under control is again paramount.

FRACTURES (BREAKS) OF THE ARM

These make up one to three percent of skiing injuries. They normally occur in a collision or fall on the outstretched hand.

Signs

Pain; deformity; swelling; considerable disability.

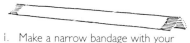

1. Make a narrow bandage with your scarf and place it across the fingers of one hand

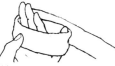

2. Wind one end once or twice around your fingers to make a loop

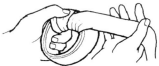

3. Bring the other end of the scarf through the loop, wind it once around the loop and pull it tight

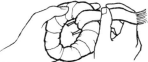

4. Working around the loop, continue passing the end through, until the whole of the scarf is used up, making a firm ring. Tuck in the end

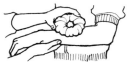

5. Place your 'scarf-ring' over the fracture site

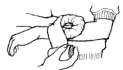

6. Place another person's scarf on the limb directly under the lower edge of your scarf-ring, make two straight turns to secure and bring the scarf up to the top of the pad again

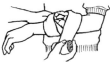

7. Continue as shown, avoiding the fracture until the pad is secure

Management

If the bone has broken the skin (compound fracture) make a 'doughnut' ring with a scarf or neckerchief (see left) and place around the fracture site to prevent anything touching the wound. Improvise a sling (see below) and go straight to a doctor for treatment.

Prevention

Again, as fractures occur in falls or collisions, be aware of your surroundings and stay in control.

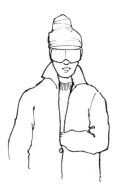

Support your injured arm in the fastening of your ski-jacket

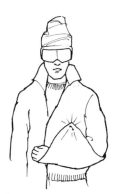

Turn up the lower edge of the casualty's ski-jacket and pin it to clothing

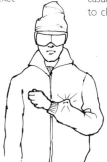

Pin the sleeve of the injured arm to clothing

OTHER INJURIES

Most other injuries to the upper limb involve sprains, cuts and bruises to the hand, wrist, arm and shoulder. They are usually undramatic and self-limiting.

Lower limb injuries are an obvious risk in skiing and account for up to seventy-two percent of all casualties. The combination of speed, hazardous surface and the long lever-arm of the ski which provides the potential for strong rotational forces applied to the leg means that the ankle, lower leg and knee are particularly vulnerable. However, due to technical improvements in the bindings, which now release more readily in a fall, and boots which are taller and stiffer and so give greater protection to the ankle, the overall rate of lower limb injuries is declining rapidly. Fractures of the lower leg have decreased by seventy-nine percent and serious ankle injuries by eighty-two percent over the past twenty years. The one glaring exception to this trend is the knee.

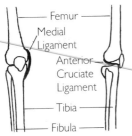

Femur
Medial Ligament
Anterior Cruciate Ligament
Tibia
Fibula

KNEE INJURIES

In contrast to this declining rate of other lower limb injuries, the rate of knee injuries has remained statistically unchanged and now accounts for twenty-five to forty percent of all skiing accidents. The knee has become the most commonly injured part of the body in skiing.

Many reasons have been advanced for this, most revolving around the influence of the bindings and boots which by saving casualties at the ankle and lower leg may simply be transferring the injurious forces up the leg to the knee. Also, the recommended binding settings for rotational toe release are designed to prevent fracture of the *tibia* (shin bone), not knee damage and the system does not react effectively to shearing forces from the side which cause the knee to buckle inwards.

These problems are compounded by the fact that the knee is anatomically predisposed to injury: it is the largest and most complex joint in the body; it lies between the two longest bones; it has to transmit movements from the hip and foot and absorb forces from the ground; it relies for its stability on the soft tissues of ligaments, joint tissue, cartilages and muscles.

The two knee structures most commonly traumatised are the *anterior cruciate ligament*, which runs through the middle

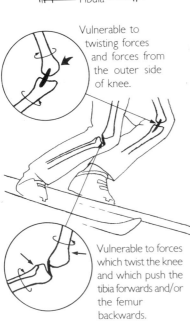

Vulnerable to twisting forces and forces from the outer side of knee.

Vulnerable to forces which twist the knee and which push the tibia forwards and/or the femur backwards.

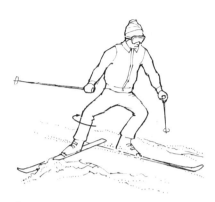

Skier wrongly leans into hill and sits too far back on turning, incorrectly weighting downhill ski. The ski's inside edge catches, it twists outwards and injures knee.

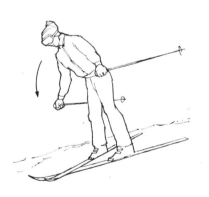

Skier stands up to rest tired muscles and leans too far forwards. Ski tips cross and skier falls forward injuring knee.

of the joint, and the *medial ligament* which lies on the outside of the joint along the inner part of the knee (see p.104). However, the other ligaments and cartilages may also be injured.

The most common mechanism of injury occurs during a turn when the skier is either wrongly sitting back on the skis or leaning into the hill and so improperly weighting the downhill ski. The turn is made off balance and the skier catches the inside edge of the downhill ski causing it to twist outwards. The skier's momentum continues taking them forwards, which accentuates the angulation of the twisting ski. This places immense strain on the cruciate and medial ligaments and severe injury is common. A similar twist on the knee happens when a wayward ski catches in deeper snow during a downhill run causing its movement to slow in relation to the rest of the body, which continues going forward. Again the wandering ski is twisted outwards and injury frequently results.

A second common injury to the knee occurs when the skier is standing erect, knees straight – usually due to fatigue – and with his/her body weight too far forward. The tips of the skis may cross or they may slow down suddenly on entering heavy snow with the result that one or both skis and boots may become fixed in relation to the upper body which continues falling forward, forcing the knee(s) backward (*hyperextension*). This puts great strain on the anterior cruciate especially and often results in isolated injury of that structure.

Signs

Pain, normally severe, although it may possibly be short lived if the anterior cruciate is injured in isolation; swelling, instability; a feeling of the knee giving way or sliding apart; strong muscle spasm.

Management

If it is simply a sprain with moderate pain and an undramatic swelling which slowly builds up over twelve to twenty-four

Four Golden Rules to Avoid Knee Injury

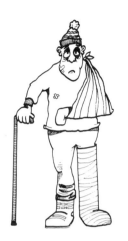

Check Fitness

hours, treat with ice packs for up to ten minutes at a time, compression in the form of a bandage, rest and elevation for twenty-four hours. After this commence gentle contractions of the thigh muscles and simple bending and straightening exercises, but continue with the ice. If the action of the knee feels in any way strange, seek medical advice. Otherwise wait for the swelling to subside and reassess pain.

If the swelling is immediate, pain severe or the knee unstable, it is likely that serious damage as been caused. Any ruptured ligament needs to be repaired as soon as possible (two weeks is the maximum delay), otherwise the torn ends retract and make direct repair impossible, so it is essential that expert medical advice is sought. If you are in a situation where this is not possible (perhaps you are uninsured or in a country not blessed with good medical facilities) then an early flight home should be considered.

Prevention

The rate of knee injuries is *the* major injury factor which we can most affect by the Fit to Ski programme. If you are quick enough to be able to react to the varying stresses and sudden obstacles of the ski slope and have the strength and endurance to do so, the opportunities for serious knee injury will be minimised. For instance, if you catch an edge and the ski begins to twist outward, if you can hone your proprioceptive systems efficiently enough to detect the unwanted rotation rapidly and instinctively correct the position of the wandering ski, then injury can be avoided. This obviously will not happen if you are too tired or too weak to react. Similarly, the hyperextension mechanism of injury is nearly always due to the skier adopting a knees straight, back erect, hips flexed position in order to give tired and aching muscles a rest. Mechanical advantage is lost in this position and what started as an attempt to allow inadequately prepared muscles to recover, ends in disaster.

Bad technique is also a major contributory factor to knee injuries, but whether it's sitting too far back, leaning into the hill on a turn, standing erect, crossing the skis or badly

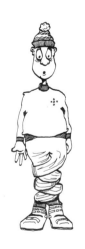

Check Technique

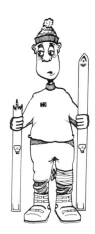

Check Bindings

executing a jump, all will be made more likely by an inappropriate and ineffective level of fitness.

You also need to be careful when skiing in fresh snow or in areas which have been inadequately pisted as this increases the likelihood of one of the skis suddenly being arrested by deeper snow; you must ensure that the bindings are set correctly for the type of terrain and your standard of ability. Care obviously has to be taken on slopes strewn with obstacles such as other skiers, trees and lift pylons, but again, quick proprioceptive reflexes and the ability of the body to carry out such reactions should enable the 'Fit to Ski' skier to cope with such difficulties.

The four golden rules for avoiding knee injuries are, therefore, check fitness, check technique, check bindings and check surroundings.

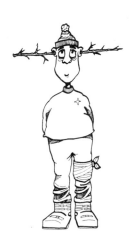

Check Surroundings

LOWER LEG FRACTURES

These now account for only eight percent of all ski trauma, representing a massive decrease over the past twenty years. The fractures are normally spiral in nature and result from excessive twisting forces to which the long lever-arm of the ski exposes the leg. They normally occur when a twisting force is coupled with a forward fall. The other major fracture is an oblique fracture which occurs when the ski becomes entrapped and the skier falls either forward, backward or to the side. With the ski ensnared, the top of the boot acts as a fulcrum and the tibia breaks at an oblique angle depending on the direction of the fall.

Signs

Intense pain; deformity; muscle spasm; immediate swelling and bruising; unable to take weight on leg; a distinct crack may be heard.

Management

Keep the injured person warm, comfortable and protected from the elements and other dangers, for instance, other skiers. Only move if strictly necessary, otherwise await rescue. If moving is unavoidable, splint leg to other leg with ski pole or broken ski.

Prevention

Prevention of this type of injury is to a great extent dependent on the bindings which should release before a fracture occurs. So it is essential that these are regularly checked and maintained. As all fractures result from falls of one type or another, good technique and skiing within your own limitations are again important. As with knee injuries, be aware of fresh or inadequately pisted snow which provides areas of relatively deeper snow in which the ski can suddenly slow.

ANKLE INJURIES

Severe ankle injures have declined in incidence even more dramatically than pure lower leg fractures of which they are a more serious variant. The mechanisms of injury are the same as for the above fractures.

Simple ankle sprains still occur in skiing although with boots rapidly improving and allowing less and less room for the ankle to turn inwards these should steadily decrease. They happen most frequently when the ski is turned inwards and the skier falls forward, a situation often encountered when attempting to master the 'snow plough' position.

More and more, however, I find myself treating sprains which have actually occurred *off* the slopes themselves with the boots removed. I think this is due to a combination of factors. When the skier removes his/her boot, especially after a long, hard day's skiing, the proprioceptive system at the ankle may have become so accustomed to having the boot's 'exo-skeleton' fitting snugly around it and so preventing much unwanted movement, that it is not ideally prepared for the twists and stresses of normal activity. The skier then goes out in to the resort which is an environment positively full of slippery sidewalks, ice covered steps and rickety stairs and goes to a restaurant or bar. By the end of the evening fatigue and perhaps alcohol have been added to the equation and the potential for trauma has been greatly increased. In years to come with rapidly progressing technical improvement making skiing inevitably safer, the short walk back to the hotel at night may become as hazardous as a day on the slopes.

For serious ankle injuries with severe pain, rapid and gross swelling and deformity, management should be the same as for lower leg fractures. For simple sprains:

Signs

Pain; swelling; tenderness on the outside of the ankle; painful, and possibly unable to bear weight on leg; movement possible but turning foot inwards causes pain.

Management

Treat with ice packs for up to fifteen minutes. Apply compression with strapping in a figure of eight fashion (see p.110) or place cotton wool around the ankle and bandage in a similar way. Rest the limb keeping it elevated above the height of the hip. After twenty four hours commence gentle exercise in elevation within the strapping or bandage, moving the ankle forwards, backwards and side to side to aid the reabsorption of the swelling. As soon as pain allows, start balancing exercises on the affected leg. Remove the strapping after forty-eight hours and reassess the problem. Strapping should be reapplied if skiing is going to be attempted. If you are in any doubt about the problem or if the injury does not appear to be healing quickly, then seek medical advice. Ironically, if there is little dramatic swelling and bruising but persistent pain, there is probably swelling encapsulated in the joint itself which is a more troublesome problem and likely to put a stop to the rest of your skiing on the holiday.

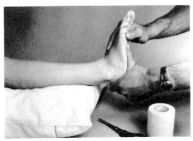

Support leg. Push ankle up and outwards. It is essential that operator and casualty try to maintain this position throughout.

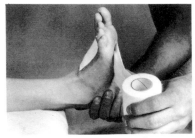

Strapping from inside to out, fix tape to top of foot just short of toes. Wrap twice around foot, with second loop nearer ankle.

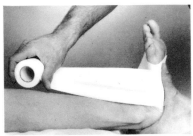

At end of second loop pull tape strongly up from outside of foot . . .

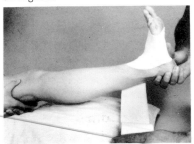

. . . and wrap around leg just above ankle.

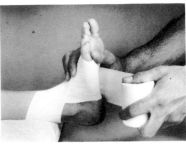

Draw strapping back down inside and under foot . . .

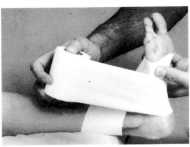

. . . and pull firmly up again from outside of foot.

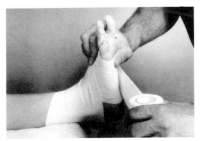

Wrap tape around ankle itself and repeat procedure round foot.

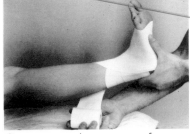

Once more apply pressure up from outside of foot and draw tape around leg overlapping first loop.

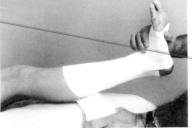

Continue tape up around leg so that strapping is in criss-cross pattern on back of calf.

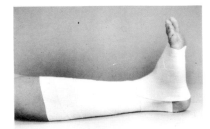

Finish at mid-calf level.

Prevention

Ensure that your boots fit correctly. If they are too loose they may increase the likelihood of injury by allowing too much movement at the ankle. This is especially true for beginners who not only have yet to acquire the good technique important in preventing most injuries, but also spend much time mastering the snow plough position in which there is a high incidence of ankle sprains. Moreover, they are not aware of how a well-fitting boot should feel – it should allow movement at the toes, only very minimal side to side movement at the ankle and the heel should be firmly gripped – so beginners must seek advice.

The smaller of the two calf muscles, especially, should be adequately stretched before skiing (see p.36). If your calf muscles consistently ache throughout the week, the boots are probably allowing too much uplift at the heel, meaning that you spend much of your time putting pressure through the balls of your feet and over-using the calf.

More than any other simple trauma, ankle injuries tend to have persistent after-effects if inadequately treated. Most of these stem from a disturbance of the balance and proprioceptive systems at the ankle. (If you have an old ankle injury compare balancing on the unaffected leg with your eyes closed with balancing on the affected leg. Often you will be much more unstable on the latter). So if you have a history of ankle problems or any weakness in that area, complete re-education of the ankle by progressive balancing exercises is essential. Even in injuries many years old, a concerted effort over one to two weeks can prove curative. The Fit to Ski programme in itself will be enough to resolve most ankle problems of this type.

KNEE BRACES

The every-increasing number of knee injuries has resulted in more and more people using a knee brace for skiing. The choice on the market in Britain gets wider every year, though it still has some way to go before it can match the diversity of the States. Knee braces are universally expensive – anything from £20 for a simple tube of neoprene to £250 for a custom-made model – and come with a host of manufacturers' claims involving strange phases like varus deformity, valgus load and axial rotation. However, the truth is that this wealth of promises is backed up by a dearth of knowledge and there is still no concrete proof that the braces work in any way other than keeping the area warm and reminding you that you have a bad knee.

To be fair to the manufacturers this is not wholly their fault as the potentially injurious forces which are experienced in skiing and against which the brace has to guard are too destructive to allow experimentation on a real knee! Studies of preserved limbs are no good as they remove the effect of the knee's major stabilisers, the muscles, and so manufacturers and the skiers alike await the development of a mechanical artificial limb which would allow valid and reliable testing.

The major constraint under which all brace manufacturers have to work is that the support must be affixed on the skin. This effectively acts as a slipping, sliding layer interposed between the brace and the underlying tissues whose movement the brace is atttempting to control. When the limb is in action it is well nigh impossible to achieve effective support of the joint by way of the skin. All manufacturers' claims about their braces being able to prevent unwanted rotational movement should therefore be viewed with a healthy degree of scepticism.

Many braces have a hinged stay either side of the knee which are claimed to prevent damaging sideways movement. This is true to a certain extent, but again because of the intervening layers of skin and brace material, the stays have to be some way from the joint they are attempting to stabilise and whether they mechanically prevent sideways movement enough to stop damage is questionable. Certainly, the longer the brace and stays are the greater inhibiting force they can exert, but also the more cumbersome they become and the more they will ultimately affect your performance.

An increasing number of manufacturers are now producing lighter braces to make them more comfortable. While these are certainly less awkward and have a decreased tendency to slip down the limb, they are also less durable and this should be taken into account especially if skiing often in an expensive brace.

Lastly, the psychological effects of having a brace should be considered. A support undoubtedly helps restore the skier's confidence in the knee, especially if major surgery has been performed, and it may allow that extra feeling of security which is the difference between an end to all sport and a guarded return to physical activity. However, there is always the danger of the skier becoming completely dependent on the brace, considering him or herself an invalid without it. Conversely, it may inculcate an unwarranted feeling of invulnerability and inspire risk taking behaviour. It must always be remembered that the brace is there to provide some help to a functionally deficient knee and the ultimate goal is to condition the knee to be able to perform adequately without it. It is not an invincible guard against all trauma.

My personal opinion is that the major effect of the braces on the market at present is in mechanically preventing bending back of the knee (hyperextension) and acting as a tactile reminder to the patient that he or she has a bad knee. This constant stimulus increases the proprioceptive awareness around the joint and heightens the reactions of the muscles to stresses and impending trauma. If this is true, and I stress it is only a personal opinion, two points should be borne in mind. Firstly, the brace should be comfortable but apply enough pressure in the correct direction to stimulate the appropriate muscles; the only way to check this is to try it on and perform some exercises which normally stress your particular condition. You will normally find that an adequate effect can be gained with a much cheaper and less complex model than is usually advocated. Secondly, in order to maximise the efficiency of these muscle reflexes to react to stresses transmitted through the brace, it is vital that you exercise with the brace on before you depart for your skiing holiday. The soft tissues of the joint and limb need to become accustomed to the feel of the brace and how to react to its varying stretches and pressures.

In summary, knee braces would appear to have a definite supporting effect on the injured knee in skiing. Whether this effect is mechanical, psychological or physiological is, however, the concern of much debate but little proof. The best advice is perhaps to try on any brace before buying it and wear the one which you feel is the most comfortable and effective for you given the demands you are going to place on it. Do not be swayed from these aims by the price or manufacturers' claims.

Sitting in a quaint, mountain top restaurant and looking down at the slopes sprinkled with bright ski suits and criss-crossed by a latticework of lifts which appear to make even the most distant peaks accessible, it is easy to forget that your skiing takes place in an environment exposed to and moulded by a harsh, tempestuous climate. Like people who grow up by the sea and develop an innate feel for its moods and ways, villagers in the mountains have a natural affinity for the climate there and can read its vagaries to a remarkable degree. With this insight comes respect. However, for the majority of us plucked for one or two weeks from the cosy convenience of city living and removed to an environment completely alien to our own, this respect is understandably often lacking. Instead, lulled into a false sense of security by the comfort of our accommodation, we often take to the slopes a dangerous and potentially fatal mixture of ignorance and naivety.

The injuries described below are not common, but are by no means rare. Everyone going skiing should be aware of them, know how to recognise and cope with them should they occur, but, most importantly, know how to prevent them.

HYPOTHERMIA

Low body temperature.

This is much more common than people think and is most frequently reported as happening to skiers stuck on a lift in bad weather, but it can actually strike anywhere under the right conditions. Certainly, anyone thinking about doing any type of ski touring should be well aware of the dangers of hypothermia.

The major climatic factors precipitating hypothermia are cold, wet and wind, with the latter being the most significant.

MILD HYPOTHERMIA

This occurs when the temperature of the body falls below 35.5°C but above 32°C.

Signs

Victim initially complains of feeling miserably cold; sluggishness; increasing lethargy; victim tends to fall behind group; shivering.

Management

The victim must be prevented from further cooling, so the major objective is to find shelter. All wet clothes should be replaced by dry ones. Do not allow the person to take a hot bath or shower as this may cause more problems, but just take them to a warm environment, such as a heated room. A hot drink is allowable, for although it will probably make the sufferer physiologically marginally cooler, the psychological benefit will outweigh this. Kept warm, dry and sheltered, the victim will warm up by him or herself.

PROFOUND HYPOTHERMIA

This occurs when body temperature falls below 32°C. It is a life-threatening emergency and must be immediately recognised and treated as such. It usually occurs on ski touring in bad weather or when someone has fallen down a crevasse or become injured and rendered immobile and the considerable heat generated by body movement is lost.

Signs

Extreme drowsiness; progressively incommunicative with slurred speech; the victim appears to be cooperating but does not in fact do so; commonly fails to protect him or herself against the cold, for instance, leaves zip of coat undone, does not pull hood up; movement becomes uncoordinated; skin is blue and cold; the breath develops a fruity smell (due to inefficient metabolism) and this is frequently the first thing others notice; incontinence of urine; shivering ceases.

Management

The primary aim of managing a victim of profound hypothermia is to keep them alive until medical help arrives. Death is normally caused by cardiac arrest, the fatal cessation of normal heartbeat. The three most common causes of death are exercising or active movement of the subject; uncomfortable or clumsy rescue; rapid rewarming.

Do not allow victim to move, for instance, trying to pull self out of a crevasse, as this will flood the person's heart with cold, acidic blood from the periphery (limbs) and possibly cause a cardiac arrest. He or she must be kept completely still and lifted onto the stretcher. Rescue must be gentle with no bumpy ride down the mountain. Insist on this, even if it means going slowly, as sudden jumps can again cause the heart to stop. Do not attempt to rewarm the victim quickly and do not give a hot drink. Prevent further heat loss by protecting from cold surroundings, replacing wet clothes with dry if possible (if not, wring them out and put back on), and protect from the wind. He or she may be cuddled by others to allow some transfer of body heat. If rescue is uncertain, rewarming can be begun centrally by placing anything that provides a gentle heat on the trunk, otherwise await rescue. *Never assume someone suffering from hypothermia is dead even if breathing and heartbeat appear absent.*

Prevention

Firstly, wear adequate clothing. It is the amount rather than the thickness of layers which is important, as air is trapped between the surfaces, warmed by the body and provides good insulation. Secondly, be aware of the weather. At any signs of incoming storms, get to shelter, do not wait for it to break before doing so. If going on a ski tour, ensure there are adequate mountain huts en route and that you know their location.

Hypothermia is especially significant as it is usually other people in the party who recognise it rather than the victim, so it is important that everyone should know what signs to look for in others.

FROSTBITE

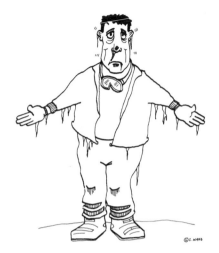

This is caused by cold which initially leads to a decrease and then a complete shut down of blood supply to the extremities resulting in the freezing of tissues, especially the toes and fingers. The nose, cheeks and ears can also be affected, although problems here are usually much less severe.

Signs

Initially pain and a feeling of cold and then a loss of all sensation. Commonly people will continuing skiing, especially if it is the toes which are affected, as they cannot feel anything and so are unaware of any problem. The affected part will also appear very pale and may eventually develop a bluish hue, but obviously in the toes and fingers these changes go unnoticed. They are, however, readily seen in the nose and ears (commonly termed 'frostnip') and changes here should be treated as a warning that a more serious problem may be occuring in the hands and feet.

Management

Rapid rewarming is the best answer. As soon as any pain or numbness is felt or whitening of the skin is observed, then the area should be treated immediately. Get to shelter if possible, if not then at least get out of the wind, and apply firm, steady pressure with a warm hand to the affected part. Do not rub the area. Fingers can be warmed very effectively by placing them in the armpits, and nose and cheeks can be relieved by blowing into hands cupped over the face. Feet can be warmed by placing them on a friend's (a good friend's!) abdomen or in the armpits. Normal colour and sensation should rapidly return and skiing can be continued. If at all possible, wet clothes, especially gloves, socks and boot insoles, should be dried before setting out again.

If, however, the affected part does not quickly regain normal appearance and feeling or if the problem appears more severe, then medical opinion should be sought immediately. If this is unavailable, as may happen when ski touring or skiing in a remote area, then every effort must be made to get to shelter as quickly as possible. The affected part should be placed in warm water which, if possible can be controlled between 42°–44°C. As the cold limb will decrease the water temperature, hot water must be added to keep the temperature constant (the limb should be removed when doing this). The water must never be sufficient to burn the tissues, so check the temperature with an unaffected part of the body. Keep the limb immersed until the skin is soft and pliable and any colour change has stopped. This may take twenty to forty minutes. The area will be painful, so care should be taken to keep the casualty as comfortable as possible. After rewarming, the part should then be dried, compressed with a bandage, elevated, rested and kept warm and clean. *If there is any doubt that this may not be possible, then re-warming should not be attempted.*

Do not rewarm if there is a possibility of refreezing as this will prove far more disastrous to the tissues.

Do not rewarm, especially the feet, if the victim is expected to be active afterwards. He or she will not be able to walk or ski and will have to be carried or towed.

Do not rub area as this may damage numb parts.
Do not use uncontrollable dry heat, for instance, placing the affected part in front of fire, as this frequently causes burning of the numbed tissues.

Prevention

Correct clothing of the periphery is essential. For hands, gloves inside mittens are best; for feet, one medium thickness, calf-length sock is usually enough but two may be worn depending upon the degree of cold and the fit of your boot. As soon as any pain is felt in fingers or toes, stop and rewarm. Do not allow to become numb. Make sure that the nose, cheeks and ears are covered with a hat and scarf on colder days and especially when skiing fast, as the wind removes heat from the thin tissues of these areas very quickly. Look out for any colour changes in your skiing partner's nose, cheeks and ears, and remember that they may indicate more serious problems elsewhere. Be aware that water is an excellent conductor of heat, so clothes should be kept as dry as possible and good waterproof clothing, especially mittens, should be worn. If skiing away from shelter, especially off piste in deep snow, a spare pair of inner gloves and socks should be taken in a waterproof bag. Metal is an even better conductor than water and in very cold conditions it will instantly cement itself to the skin at the lightest touch. Therefore, in extreme conditions metal objects such as zips and ski bindings should not be touched with bare skin.

Frostbite is made more likely if the blood supply to the periphery is additionally impeded by factors other than cold. The two major culprits are hypothermia and tight-fitting boots. Therefore, ensure that all steps to prevent hypothermia are taken (p. 116) and that boots are not too restrictive (or made to be because of too thick socks), especially around the top of the ankle. Be aware of the fact that feet swell during exercise and this may make boots tighter than they would normally feel.

ARCTIC WILLY

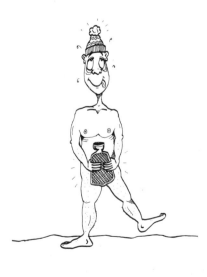

This is a form of frostbite, mercifully mild, which affects the male genitalia. It is not widely recognised, the above diagnostic term only recently being coined, though personally I would have preferred the more alliterative and less geographically exclusive 'Chilly Willy'. A natural reticence has lead to an under-reporting of cases, but it is nonetheless an uncomfortable and disquieting condition. Inadequate clothing is the most common cause, especially the wearing of trousers which are too tight or boxer shorts which allow the penis to pop out and touch the cold metal zip.

Signs

Pain on passing water; numbness and redness, particularly of the foreskin; possible pain; swelling may appear later.

Management

Given the lack of reports of this condition, management is a difficult area. The standard treatment of frostbite – rapidly rewarming the affect parts in a bowl of warm water at 42°C–44°C – would in these circumstances demand a peculiarly shaped bowl or considerable gymnastic talent. A warm and personal shower is the best alternative. The late actor, David Niven, sustained probably the most celebrated case of Arctic Willy while skiing in the Italian Alps during the shooting of *The Pink Panther*. He describes how the Italian guides administered the standard local treatment of immersing his 'pale blue acorn' into a glass of neat whisky. This proved painful but curative and also managed to give a whole new meaning to the drink 'scotch on the rocks'.

Prevention

Prevention is really the only answer. Loose fitting, windproof trousers with long johns in colder weather should be worn. As soon as any discomfort or numbness is felt, stop, rewarm and cross your fingers!

SKI BOOT FOOT SYNDROME

This is a tender swelling of the skin of the foot, predominantly affecting the sole. It results from the feet being exercised for long periods at a time in very well-insulated, plastic ski boots. The insoles become soaked with moisture from sweat and their excellent thermal insulating properties produce a closed and saturated mini-environment which gradually softens and waterlogs the skin. The condition has also been reported as happening to people wearing moon boots for the long coach and sea journey to and from the resort.

Signs

The skin is swollen, tender, soft, white and wrinkled.

Management

Removal of footwear and cleaning and drying feet will produce overnight resolution of the symptoms. However, if circumstances are repeated, symptoms do tend to recur. If it is becoming a problem it may be worth skiing down to your accommodation at lunchtime and removing the boots for an hour or so. If this is impractical, a comfortably warm restaurant will suffice, but make sure it is actually hot inside and not just warm compared to the temperature outside. If the air is cold it will simply chill or even freeze the sweat on the insoles.

Prevention

There is no real solution apart from trying to avoid wearing boots continuously for long periods and making sure the insoles are cleaned and dried as often as possible. Wearing non-synthetic socks will probably help, and lightly dusting the feet with talcum powder may prove beneficial. This condition will also unfortunately predispose you to fungal infections such as athelete's foot and these must be looked out for.

SNOW BLINDNESS

This is a degree of visual impairment, some or possibly all of which may remain permanently. It is caused by the increased presence of ultra-violet light in the atmosphere; the thinner atmosphere of the mountains absorbs less UV than normal and there is greater reflection from surroundings. It is especially important to realise that snow blindness symptoms do not normally appear until some time after exposure and so the victim may be unaware at the time of doing any damage.

Signs

Pain in the eyes, frequently intense; feeling that eyes are full of sand or pepper; red and watering eyes; sensitivity to light.

Management

Bathe eyes in cold water, wear sunglasses if during day and seek medical advice.

Prevention

Wear good sunglasses with one hundred percent ultraviolet absorption, preferably with sides, or goggles and do not take them off at any time whilst on the slopes. Even ten minutes exposure can cause irreversible damage.

SUNBURN

The sun in the thin air of the mountains is extremely strong. Its burning effect on the skin is not equivalent to the Mediterranean on a sunny day, more the scorching heat of the Sahara. Moreover, it is reflected from the surrounding snow and ice on to every nook and cranny of exposed skin, from ear lobes to nostrils, from under the chin to the top of the scalp. If you normally tan quickly and well and usually make do with a low factor lotion, it is completely irrelevant. This is not a comparable environment to the seaside. Use factor 15 or block out. It is still possible to get a tan through the week: even the very high factors allow enough ultraviolet through during the day to enable everyone to return home with that tell-tale healthy glow. You certainly won't be doing that, however, if you burn your face to blistering on the first day by underestimating the sun's powers. Apart from ruining the skiing holiday this can scar victims permanently.

Signs

Redness; stinging; possible blistering

Management

If only mild, bathe gently with cold water or spread with cool lotion, preferably moisturiser and keep clean and out of sunlight. If severe, go to the doctor. Second and occasionally third degree burns are a real possibility in the mountains. Whatever the temptation, do *not* burst blisters.

Prevention

Sunburn is entirely preventable. It only arises as a result of ignorance and vanity. The clear message is to cover up. Smother your exposed skin with a very high factor lotion (at least 15), your nose and ears with block out. If you are fair and burn easily, use block out all over. Reapply often (at least every two hours), more if you are perspiring heavily or if it is a very sunny day. Be sensible and there is no reason why you should suffer.

As in most things, children need particular care when skiing, so it is important to follow these simple guidelines:

1   They are more vulnerable to cold, though, in many cases, less likely to mention it than adults, so make sure they are wrapped up in an adequate amount of layers paying special attention to the extremities.

2   It is essential that the bindings are set at the right strength. Let the ski shop do this. However, there does appear to be a high rate of binding failure in children and some authors have recommended that until more reliable systems are available for children, the heel piece should be set according to the standard scale but the toe mechanism be set as loose as possible without causing release during normal skiing.

3   Children should *always* wear crash helmets when skiing. Their skulls are not as tough as adults and therefore more susceptible to injury.

4   They also seem to be more affected by lack of regular food and fluid, so make sure they eat and drink well and regularly.

5   Finally, many kids appear to have no fear and put us trembling adults to shame. Keep an eye on them and make sure they don't go whizzing into beginners or shooting off piste when your back is turned.

BEFORE SKIING

1 Breakfast, including cereal, bread or toast and drink.

2 Check weather.

3 If touring, check weather reports, route and position of huts.

4 Apply high factor sun lotion to exposed areas and blockout to nose, ears and lips.

5 Quick stretching exercises in room.

6 Take hat and scarf, money, piste map, sun lotion and blockout, snacks for rest periods, sunglasses, goggles in bad weather and, if needed, spare inner gloves and socks in waterproof bag.

7 Check bindings.

8 Check skis, especially edges and braking mechanism.

9 Quick warm up exercises on slope.

DURING SKIING

10 Don't take sunglasses off on slope.

11 Grip pole outside strap.

12 Ski within own limitations and ignore peer pressure.

13 Check speed.

14 Be aware of terrain, especially worn and icy patches, rocky areas and roots of trees.

15 Be aware of other skiers and give them room.

16 Take constant note of weather and take shelter when necessary. Do not be loath to stop for the day if weather is really unpleasant.

17   Rest when tired and be especially careful at the end of the morning and afternoon sessions.

18   Do not skip lunch.

19   Have regular snacks and drinks.

20   Any cold or numbness, especially in extremities, or feelings of being miserably cold, whether you or your partner, then get to shelter and warm up immediately.

21   Do not drink any alcohol.

AFTER SKIING

22   Stretch off.

23   Dry and clean clothes, especially boot insoles and mittens and inners.

24   Pay special attention to condition of skin of feet and any sunburnt areas.

25   Rest and eat well, including at least one of the following: potatoes, rice, bread, pasta.

26   Have fun but watch the slippery walk home.